Jürgen Gießing, Michael Fröhlich & Peter Preuss
(Editors)

Current Results of Strength Training Research
An empirical and theoretical Approach

Bibliografische Information Der Deutschen Bibliothek
Die Deutsche Bibliothek verzeichnet diese Publikation in der Deutschen Nationalbibliografie; detaillierte bibliografische Daten sind im Internet über http://dnb.ddb.de abrufbar.
1. Aufl. - Göttingen : Cuvillier, 2005
ISBN 3-86537-568-5

Umschlaggestaltung
KLEIN - Mediengestaltung GdbR
Detzelstraße 6
D-66386 St. Ingbert

Nonnenstieg 8, 37075 Göttingen
Telefon: 0551-54724-0
Telefax: 0551-54724-21
www.cuvillier.de

1. Auflage, 2005
Gedruckt auf säurefreiem Papier

ISBN 3-86537-568-5

Foreword by Prof. Dr. Dietmar Schmidtbleicher

Sport science has progressed considerably in recent years and many high-performance athletes, coaches and support staff have gone on record to say that sport science plays a key role in optimizing training and performance.
If this is true in general, for the topic of strength and strength training the increase of knowledge during the last 25 years was tremendous. Therefore coaches, athletes and managers of fitness and sports need to be well informed about the benefits of this specific area.
With good coaching and support over many years an athlete may be trained to near perfection before and during a major event. And the same is true for normal sportsmen und even housewives. The only difference exists in the intensities and volumes of workouts.
New knowledge in sport science offers a wide range becoming increasingly aware of the importance of the inclusion of strength and conditioning in the training programmes.
Avoidance of injury and optimum physical preparation are crucial to ensure sustainable success in high performance sports as well as in health cure. Posture, coordination, balance, eccentric control, agility, core strength and stability and important for all factors: strength, speed and their product power, all contribute to sports performance.
This collection of new knowledge enables specialists in sports, medical doctors, physical education teachers and students as well as coaches and athletes to discover a new insight in the topic of strength and strength training.

Frankfurt/Main, September 2005

Prof. Dr. Dietmar Schmidtbleicher

Preface

> "The ability to generate force has fascinated humankind throughout most of recorded history. Not only have great feats of strength intrigued people´s imagination, but a sufficient level of muscular strength was important for survival." (American College of Sports Medicine, 2002, p.364)

This book presents current results of strength training research as well as theoretical concepts of strength training. It deals with a variety of different aspects of strength training in order to provide the reader with as much information as possible.

Among others, these topics include single-set versus multiple-set training, fundamental definitions of decisive training parameters, the methodology of strength training, post-exhaustion, testing strength and other related topics. These topics are being studied all over the world. This is the reason why an international approach was chosen for this book. Each article presents the conclusions and views of the respective author(s) which are meant to contribute to the discourse on the several aspects of strength training and which might be interesting for athletes, coaches as well as for therapists and scholars.

Acknowledgements

We would like to thank the authors for supplying the articles for this book. We also thank Mr. Markus Klein for his efforts in the production (cover design and proofreading) and Dr. Andrea Pieter for proofreading.

We acknowledge the important contributions to this book by each of our esteemed colleagues. It was really an international team effort by a group of scholars who have worked tirelessly in this area of study for years.

Marburg, Saarbrücken and Bonn, September 2005 the editors

Topic

JÜRGEN GIEßING, PETER PREUSS, ANDREAS GREIWING, SVEN GOEBEL, ANDREAS MÜLLER, ALEXANDER SCHISCHEK & ANIKA STEPHAN

Fundamental definitions of decisive training parameters of single-set training and multiple-set training for muscle hypertrophy

Keywords: single-set training, multiple-set training, hypertrophy, training intensity, strength training parameters

Introduction

One aspect of strength training that is being discussed controversially is the optimal amount of training volume necessary for inducing maximum increases in muscle strength and hypertrophy. Especially the concept of single-set training has been suggested to be a practical alternative to multiple-set training. Another factor that is directly related to this aspect is the degree of training intensity at which a set is carried out. The term *training intensity* is defined as "the possible momentary muscular effort being exerted" (Mentzer, 1996, p. 46).

When comparing the results of various studies it becomes obvious that there are various different definitions of single-set training. Single-set training has either been defined as

- one set of eight to ten repetitions to failure per muscle group (Schlumberger & Schmidtbleicher, 1999, p. 9) or
- as one set per exercise which implies that several exercises may be done per muscle group (Gießing, 2004).

In many important publications single-set training is not mentioned at all (Hollmann, Hettinger, & Strüder, 2000; Marées, 2002; Martin, Carl, & Lehnertz, 1993; Weineck, 2000). Hohmann, Lames & Letzelter (2002, p. 80) mention single-set training as a training method in strength training but do not offer a definition.

Fleck & Kraemer (2004, p. 188) describe single-set training as "performance of each exercise for one set [...] using heavy resistances and a few repetitions per set with a 5-minute rest between exercises". The American College of

Sports Medicine suggests one set of eight to ten repetitions to failure for recreational athletes who train with an emphasis on improving their health whereas elderly persons should rather keep their repetitions in the range between ten and 15 and should use lighter weights (ACSM, 1998, p. 983). Wilmore & Costill (2004, p. 107) mention single-set training as one of many strength training methods but do not give any information concerning the parameters number of repetitions, relative intensity (percentage of 1-RM) or training intensity. Boeckh-Behrens & Buskies (2000, p. 71) refer to single-set training as "one set per exercise or one set per muscle group respectively" and state that sets do not have to be carried to failure as it is often suggested as opposed to Philipp (1999, p. 31) who suggests that each set should be taken to failure or even beyond.

This shows that there exists considerable inconsistency concerning the definitions of the term single-set training itself and furthermore the degree of training intensity necessary in order to successfully apply this training method. This inconsistency is surprising especially considering the fact that single-set training is common in both recreational and competitive sports (Ebben & Blackard, 2001, p. 57).

The relevance of the parameter training intensity

The necessary training intensity is an aspect that has often been neglected when discussing training parameters applied in single-set training.

Therefore, Heiduk, Preuss & Steinhöfer (2002) differentiated between single-set training (SST) and high-intensity training (HIT) as an intense version of single-set training. They further differentiated between "high-volume training" (HVT) and "low-volume training" (LVT) defining LVT as a training volume of one ore two sets per exercise and HVT as at least three sets per exercise. According to their definition SST and HIT are forms of LVT whereas multiple-set training (MST) has to be considered HVT (see figure 1).

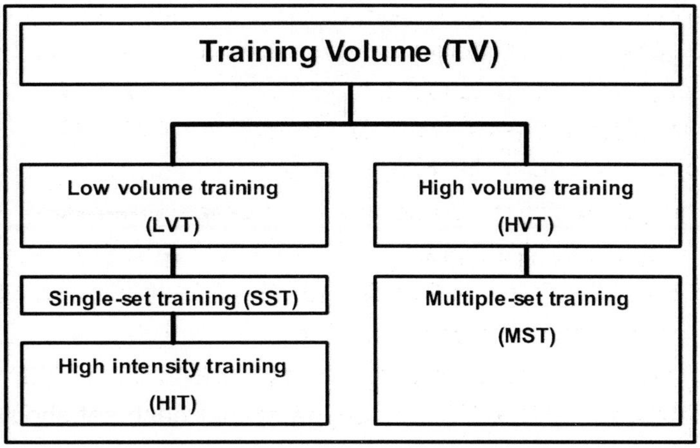

Figure 1: Differentiation of training volume (cf. Heiduk et al., 2002).

The factor training intensity should be dealt with in more detail since the publications by Zatsiorsky (1996), Buskies (1999a) and Boeckh-Behrens & Buskies (2000) imply that a distinction in SST and HIT does not cover all the necessary differentiations of this factor.

Tidow (1999, p. 52) suggests that hypertrophy training requires a compromise between the degree of tension and the time under tension at a given percentage of 1-RM. When training volume is calculated as *number of sets x number of repetitions x load,* the *time under tension* (TUT) is not included in the calculation. It has often been suggested by proponents of single-set training that this factor must not be ignored (Brzycki, 1995; Kieser, 1998). Remmert, Schischek, Zamhöfer and Ferrauti (2005) proved in their HIT study that TUT can be a useful parameter for the evaluation and regulation of strength training programs.

It can be summed up that there is a need to clarify the following aspects of SST and MST for muscle hypertrophy training:

- the controversy of SST either meaning one set per exercise or one set per muscle (group),
- the need to differentiate between different degrees of training intensity and
- repetition speed in terms of TUT.

Empirical studies

Recent meta-analyses have compared the results of SST to those of MST (Carpinelli, 2002; Peterson, Rhea, & Alvar, 2004; Rhea, Alvar, Ball, & Burkett, 2002; Rhea, Alvar, Burkett, & Ball, 2003; Winett, 2004; Wolfe, LeMura, & Cole, 2004). An analysis of the studies that these meta-analyses were based on shows that the inconsistency mentioned before is also apparent when comparing the different study designs.

Number of exercises per muscle group

Table 1 shows that only the studies by Borst et al. (2001), Capen (1956), Jacobson (1986), Kramer et al. (1997), Pollock et al. (1993), Schlumberger, Stec and Schmidtbleicher (2001) and Starkey et al. (1996) studied the results of one exercise per muscle group. The training programs in the studies by Borst et al. (2001) and Schlumberger et al. (2001) represent whole-body training programs.

Table 1: Number of exercises per muscle group in empirical SST studies

exercises per muscle group	study
1 exercise	Borst et al. (2001), Capen (1956), Jacobson (1986), Kramer et al. (1997), Pollock et al. (1993), Schlumberger et al. (2001), Starkey et al. (1996)
1 and > 1 exercise	Hass, Garzarella, de Hoyos and Pollock (2000), Kraemer (1997), Marx et al. (2001), Paulsen, Myklestad and Raastad (2003), Reid, Yeather and Ullrich (1987), Rhea, Alvar, Ball and Burkett (2002), Sanborn et al. (2000), Silvester, Stiggins, McGown and Bryce (1981), Stowers et al. (1983)
> 1 exercise	Ostrowski, Wilson, Weatherby, Murphy and Lyttle (1997)
no data	Berger (1962), De Hoyos et al. (1997), De Hoyos et al. (1998), Hass, Garzarella, De Hoyos and Pollock (1998)

This overview shows that defining SST as one set of eight to ten repetitions to failure per muscle group (Schlumberger & Schmidtbleicher, 1999, p. 9) does not cover the whole variety in which SST is used. Another problem is that many exercises do not only stress one muscle group directly but do also stress other muscle groups indirectly. Every multiple-joint exercise for the upper body does not only involve the target muscle but also smaller muscles contracting synergistically. It is not possible to perform bench presses without contracting muscles of the shoulder and the triceps. If one wanted to actually restrict training volume to one exercise per muscle group, multiple-joint exercise could not be used at all. This would be the exact opposite of what the ACSM recommends:

> "It is recommended that both exercise types be included in a resistance training program with emphasis on multiple-joint exercises for maximizing muscle strength and closed kinetic chain movement capabilities in novice, intermediate, and advanced individuals." (ACSM, 2002, p. 368)

Fleck & Kraemer (2004, p. 159) also recommend using multiple-joint exercises since most activities of daily living in general and most sports activities in particular consist of multiple-joint movements.

Degrees of training intensity (DTI)

Training intensity can be rated by the criteria for terminating a set. There are four degrees of training intensity (DTI):

(1) Reaching a certain number of repetitions that does *not* represent the repetition maximum (nRM),

(2) the repetition maximum (RM),

(3) the point of momentary muscular failure (PMF),

(4) training beyond the point of momentary muscular failure (PMF+) by applying high-intensity training methods (HITM) like forced repetitions, cheating, drop sets etc. This methodical approach provides the athlete with an opportunity maximise training intensity. HITM are sometimes also referred to as high-intensity techniques or systems (Fleck & Kraemer, 2004, pp. 187-206).

Looking at the empirical studies the most commonly used DTI for multiple-set training is the RM and for single-set training it is the PMF (see table 2).

Table 2: Degrees of training intensity of empirical studies concerning SST and MST. Studies using different degrees of training intensity are highlighted in Italics

	SST	MST
nRM		*Kramer et al. (1997), Marx et al. (2001), Messier and Dill (1985), Stone, Johnson and Carter (1979)*
RM	Berger (1962), Capen (1956), Leighton, Holmes, Benson, Wooten and Schmerer (1967), Paulsen et al. (2003), Reid et al. (1987), Rhea et al. (2002), Schlumberger et al. (2001)	Borst et al. (2001), De Hoyos et al. (1998), De Hoyos et al. (1997), Hass et al. (1998), Hass et al. (2000), Ostrowski et al. (1997), Starkey et al. (1996) *Coleman (1977), Jacobson (1986), Kraemer (1997, study 2, 3 and 4), Kraemer et al. (2000), Sanborn et al. (2000), Silvester et al. (1981), Stowers et al. (1983)*
PMF	Borst et al. (2001), De Hoyos et al. (1998), De Hoyos et al. (1997), Hass et al. (1998), Hass et al. (2000), Ostrowski et al. (1997), Starkey et al. (1996) *Coleman (1977), Kraemer et al. (2000), Kramer et al. (1997), Marx et al. (2001), Messier and Dill (1985), Sanborn et al. (2000), Silvester et al. (1981), Stone, Johnson and Carter (1979), Stowers et al. (1983)*	Stowers et al. (1983)
PMF+	Pollock et al. (1993) *Kraemer (1997, study 2, 3 and 4), Jacobson (1986)*	

The difference between RM and PMF is not trivial. Quotes by Fleck and Kraemer (2004) show that there seems to be a problem distinguishing between RM and PMF:

> „A repetition maximum or RM is the maximal number of repetitions per set that can be performed with proper lifting technique using a given resistance. Thus, a set at a certain RM implies that the set is performed to momentary voluntary fatigue." (Fleck & Kraemer, 2004, p. 5)

Later they state:

> „An exhaustion set is a set performed until no further complete repetitions with good exercise technique can be completed. Synonymous with exhaustion sets are the terms carrying sets to volitional fatigue, sets to failure, and sets to concentric failure. ... The use of a repetition maximum (RM) or an RM training zone (i.e., 4-6RM) in a training program indicates that sets were carried to exhaustion." (Fleck & Kraemer, 2004, p. 196)

Obviously the terms *concentric failure* and *momentary voluntary failure* are not clearly defined. The difference between the RM and the PMF is that the RM means that the set is terminated after the final repetition has been completed in good form (Baechle, Earle, & Wathen, 2000, p. 406; Müller, 2003, p. 135; Tan, 1999, p. 291) whereas the PMF means that once the RM has been reached another repetition is attempted but not completed. Therefore the last repetition is the failed repetition.

A part of the studies mentioned in table 2 (highlighted in Italics; Coleman, 1977; Jacobson, 1986; Kraemer, 1997; Kraemer et al., 2000; Kramer et al., 1997; Marx et al., 2001; Messier & Dill, 1985; Sanborn et al., 2000; Stone et al., 1979; Stowers et al., 1983) used different degrees of training intensity to compare SST and MST. Due to the varied training volume these studies only provide clues concerning the possible outcomes of different degrees of training intensity.

A different approach of dealing with different degrees of training intensity was shown by Buskies (1999b) and his "moderate strength training". Training sets will be terminated at a certain rating of perceived exertion ranging from "moderate" to "heavy", thereby using nRMs for all sets.

Repetition speed in terms of time under tension (TUT)

In most of the studies the recent meta-analyses are based on there is no information about repetition speed or TUT as table 3 shows:

*Table 3: Repetition speed in empirical SST studies (*3 phases of a repetition: concentric phase, isometric phase, eccentric phase)*

no/insufficient data	TUT per repetition concentric/isometric/eccentric* [sec]	
Berger (1962), Capen (1956), De Hoyos et al. (1997), De Hoyos et al. (1998), Hass et al. (1998), Jacobson (1986), Kramer et al. (1997), Leighton et al. (1967), Ostrowski et al. (1997), Paulsen et al. (2003), Reid et al. (1987), Rhea, Alvar et al. (2002), Sanborn et al. (2000), Schlumberger et al. (2001), Silvester et al. (1981), Stowers et al. (1983)	Coleman (1977), Kraemer (1997), Kraemer (2000), Kramer (1997), Pollock et al. (1993), Stone et al. (1979)	2/1/4
	Hass et al. (2000), Marx et al. (2001), Starkey et al. (1996)	2/0/4
	Borst et al. (2001)	2/0/3

For SST a TUT of five to seven seconds per repetition with an emphasis on the eccentric phase seems to be most common. Many authors suggest that a slow and controlled repetition speed has a positive effect on muscle hypertrophy because of

- a larger exhaustion of energy storages,
- a stronger muscle fiber activation (Hartmann & Tünnemann, 1993, p. 56; Hemmling, 1994, pp. 21-22; Kelso, 2000, p. 65; Westcott, 1995, p. 77; Westcott et al., 2001, p. 155) and
- a longer time under tension (Hollmann & Hettinger, 1990, p. 235).

A too fast execution of repetitions and too much momentum are believed to be factors which reduce the hypertrophy stimulus and might lead to injuries (Brzycki, 1995; Westcott et al., 2001).
Several authors have studied the effects of varied worl loads on muscular performance (Almasbakk & Hoff, 1996; Jones, Bishop, Hunter, & Fleisig, 2001; McBride, Triplett-McBride, Davie, & Newton, 2002; Moss, Refsnes, Abildgaard, Nicolaysen, & Jensen, 1997; Schlumberger, 2000; Schlumberger & Schmidtbleicher, 2001; Schlumberger, Wirth, Liu, Steinacker, & Schmidtbleicher, 2003; Schmidtbleicher, 1980; Tidow & Wiemann, 1993; Toji, Suei, & Kaneko, 1997; Wilson, Newton, Murphy, & Humphries, 1993), however, none of the studies concentrated on training to failure for muscular hypertrophy using different repetition speeds and keeping the other training parameters the same.
Pereira & Gomes (2003) give an overview on studies applying different repetition speeds and find contradictory results:

> "Although both slow and fast training improved performance, faster training showed some advantages in quantity and magnitude of training effects" (Morrissey, Harman, Frykman, & Han, 1998, p. 221).

It has to be stated that study results concerning the effects of different repetition speeds are too inconsistent and even contradictory to draw a final conclusion, however, it is possible give fundamental definitions concerning the parameters *training volume* and *degrees of training intensity*.

Fundamental definitions

Based on the considerations explained above the following conclusions concerning definitions and specifications of single-set and multiple-set training are to be drawn (see table 4):

(1) **Single-set training (SST)** means that one set per exercise is performed which includes the possibility of performing more than one exercise per muscle group.

(2) **Multiple-set training (MST)** means two or more sets per exercise are performed. The break between sets takes at least 30 seconds (cf. Kraemer, 2002, p. 51).

(3) There are four different **degrees of training intensity**: The non repetition maximum (nRM), the repetition maximum (RM), the point of mo-

mentary muscular failure (PMF) and the point of momentary muscular failure plus high-intensity training methods (PMF+).

Table 4: Overview of training volumes and degrees of training intensity

training volumes	
SST	single-set training One set per exercise is performed which includes the possibility of performing more than one exercise per muscle group.
HIT	high-intensity training Single-set training using HITM in order to train beyond concentric failure. One or more exercises per muscle group could be performed.
LVT	low-volume training One or two sets per exercise and only few sets per muscle group. One ore more exercises per muscle group may be performed.
MST	multiple-set training Two or more sets per exercise with a break of at least 30 seconds between two sets of the same exercise. One ore more exercises per muscle group may be performed.
HVT	high-volume training Multiple-set training consisting of three or more sets per exercise and several exercises per muscle group.
degrees of training intensity (DTI)	
nRM	non repetition maximum Terminating a set at a fixed number of repetitions or a certain rate of perceived exertion whereas additional repetitions are possible.
RM	repetition maximum Terminating a set after the final repetition that can be completed in proper form.
PMF	point of momentary muscular failure Terminating a set when concentric failure has been reached, i. e. the final repetition can not be fully completed due to fatigue.
PMF+	point of momentary muscular failure plus HITM Training beyond failure by applying high-intensity training methods (HITM) like forced repetitions, drop set, cheating etc.

Conclusions

The definitions given above make it possible to distinguish between several degrees of training intensities which undeniably is an important factor in muscle hypertrophy training. It could be shown that the term single-set training has to be defined a one set *per exercise* which means that in a single-set training program several exercises may be performed for the same muscle group. Single-set training as well as multiple-set training can be performed at different degrees of training intensity. If high-intensity training methods are applied in single-set training, this version of SST is called high-intensity training (HIT). In rehabilitation and recreational training sets may be terminated at an nRM whereas in muscle hypertrophy training higher degrees of training intensity (RM, PMF or even PMF+) are generally applied.

If high degrees of of training intensity are applied, single-set training has been shown to be at least equally effective for muscle hypertrophy than multiple-set training at lower levels of training intensity (Gießing, 2003; Hass et al., 2000; Heiduk et al., 2002; Pollock, 1998). One training parameter that can still not be defined properly is the optimal repetition speed or TUT for muscle hypertrophy training. Calculating training volume by simply multiplying *number of sets x number of repetitions x load* does not consider TUT which should be included in the calculation in order to study its relevance for inducing muscular hypertrophy. Several studies have compared the results of SST to those of MST, however, training volume is only one of many strength training parameters (see figure 2).

Time under tension (TUT) sets x repetitions x duration of repetitions	**Power** p = w / t	**Total Force (TF)** sets x repetitions x load
Intensity • intensity (% 1-RM) • degrees of training intensity (DTI) • repetition speed	**Training volume (TV)** • sets • repetitions	**Training Interval** • rest between sets and repetitions
Selection and Order of Exercises • muscle group • training session	**Form of Contraction**	**Training Frequency**

Figure 2: Profile of strength training parameters.

Analysing the results of studies that concentrate on the relevance of a certain training parameter, there needs to be as much information as possible regarding the other strength training parameters. Several questions concerning the results of SST to those of MST remain unanswered:

It has yet to be found out which effects changing TUT and/or DTI - while keeping the other training parameters the same - has on the following factors:

- muscle hypertrophy,
- muscle fibre activation,
- lactate kinetics,
- hormonal parameters and
- rating of perceived exertion.

References

ACSM. (1998). American College of Sports Medicine Position Stand. The recommended quantity and quality of exercise for developing and maintaining cardiorespiratory and muscular fitness, and flexibility in healthy adults. *Medicine & Science in Sports & Exercise, 30*(6), 975-991.

ACSM. (2002). American College of Sports Medicine Position Stand. Progression models in resistance training for healthy adults. *Medicine & Science in Sports & Exercise, 34*(2), 364-380.

Almasbakk, B., & Hoff, J. (1996). Coordination, the determinant of velocity specificity? *Journal of Applied Physiology, 81*(5), 2046-2052.

Baechle, T. R., Earle, R., & Wathen, D. (2000). Resistance training. In T. R. Baechle & R. Earle (Eds.), *Essentials of strength training and conditioning* (pp. 395-425). Champaign, IL: Human Kinetics.

Berger, R. A. (1962). Effect of varied weight training programs on strength. *Research quarterly for exercise and sport, 33*(2), 168-181.

Boeckh-Behrens, W.-U., & Buskies, W. (2000). *Fitness-Krafttraining [Fitness strength training]* (1st ed.). Reinbek bei Hamburg: Rowohlt.

Borst, S. E., De Hoyos, D. V., Garzarella, L., Vincent, K., Pollock, B. H., Lowenthal, D. T., et al. (2001). Effects of resistance training on insulin-like growth factor-I and IGF binding proteins. *Medicine & Science in Sports & Exercise, 33*(4), 648-653.

Brzycki, M. (1995). *A practical approach to strength training* (3rd ed.). Lincolnwood, IL: Masters Press.

Buskies, W. (1999a). Sanftes Krafttraining nach dem subjektiven Belastungsempfinden versus Training bis zur muskulären Ausbelastung [Moderate strength training regulated by RPE versus training until muscle exhaustion]. *Deutsche Zeitschrift für Sportmedizin, 50*(10), 316-320.

Buskies, W. (1999b). *Sanftes Krafttraining. Unter besonderer Berücksichtigung des subjektiven Belastungsempfindens [Moderate strength training. Under special consideration of the rate of perceived exertion]*. Köln: Sport und Buch Strauß.

Capen, E. K. (1956). Study of four programs of heavy resistance exercises for development of muscular strength. *Research Quarterly, 27*(2), 132-142.

Carpinelli, R. N. (2002). Berger in retrospect: effect of varied weight training programmes on strength. *British Journal of Sports Medicine, 36*(3), 319-324.

Coleman, A. E. (1977). Nautilus vs universal gym strength training in adult males. *American Corrective Therapy Journal, 31*(4), 103-107.

De Hoyos, D., Abe, T., Garzarella, L., Hass, C., Nordman, M., & Pollock, M. L. (1998). Effects of 6 months of high- or low-volume resistance training on muscular strength and endurance. *Medicine & Science in Sports & Exercise, 30*(5), S165.

De Hoyos, D., Herring, D., Garzarella, L., Werber, G., Brechue, W. F., & Pollock, M. L. (1997). Effect of strength training volume on the development of strength and power in adolescent tennis players. *Medicine & Science in Sports & Exercise, 30*(5), S164.

Ebben, W. P., & Blackard, D. O. (2001). Strength and conditioning practices of National Football League strength and conditioning coaches. *Journal of Strength and Conditioning Research, 15*(1), 48-58.

Fleck, S. J., & Kraemer, W. J. (2004). *Designing resistance training programs* (3rd ed.). Champaign, IL: Human Kinetics.

Gießing, J. (2003). Training for muscular hypertrophy: A comparison of high and low-volume approaches. *International Journal of Physical Education, 15*(1), 27-32.

Gießing, J. (2004). *1 Satz Training - Ein wissenschaftlich fundiertes Konzept für schnellstmöglichen Muskelaufbau im Bodybuilding [Single-set training. A concept for rapid muscle gains based on scientific findings]* (1st ed.). Arnsberg: Novagenics.

Hartmann, J., & Tünnemann, H. (1993). *Modernes Krafttraining [Modern strength training]*. Berlin: Ullstein.

Hass, C. J., Garzarella, L., De Hoyos, D., & Pollock, M. L. (1998). Effects of training volume on strength and endurance in experienced resistance trained adults. *Medicine & Science in Sports & Exercise, 30*(5), S115.

Hass, C. J., Garzarella, L., de Hoyos, D., & Pollock, M. L. (2000). Single versus multiple sets in long-term recreational weightlifters. *Medicine & Science in Sports & Exercise, 32*(1), 235-242.

Heiduk, R., Preuss, P., & Steinhöfer, D. (2002). Die optimale Satzzahl im Krafttraining: Einsatz- versus Mehrsatz-Training [The optimal number of sets: single-set versus multiple-set training]. *Leistungssport, 32*(4), 4-13.

Hemmling, G. (1994). *Anpassungen des neuromuskulären Systems an eine neuentwickelte Trainingsmethode [Adaptations of the neuromuscular systems to a newly developed training method]*. Köln: Sport und Buch Strauß.

Hohmann, A., Lames, M., & Letzelter, M. (2002). *Einführung in die Trainingswissenschaft [Introduction in training science]* (1st ed.). Wiebelsheim: Limpert.

Hollmann, W., & Hettinger, T. (1990). *Sportmedizin - Arbeits und Trainingsgrundlagen [Sports medicine - labour and training fundamentals]* (3rd ed.). Stuttgart, New York: Schattauer.

Hollmann, W., Hettinger, T., & Strüder, H. (2000). *Sportmedizin - Grundlagen für Arbeit, Training und Präventivmedizin [Sports medicine - fundamentals of labour, training and prevention medicine]* (4th ed.). Stuttgart, New York: Schattauer.

Jacobson, B. H. (1986). A comparison of two progressive weight training techniques on knee extensor strength. *Athletic Training, 21*(4), 315-318, 390.

Jones, K., Bishop, P., Hunter, G., & Fleisig, G. (2001). The effects of varying resistance-training loads on intermediate- and high-velocity-specific adaptations. *Journal of Strength and Conditioning Research, 15*(3), 349-356.

Kelso, T. (2000). The basics of muscle contraction: implications for strength training. In M. Brzycki (Ed.), *Maximize your training: insights from leading strength and fitness professionals* (pp. 35-80). Lincolnwood, IL: Master Press.

Kieser, W. (1998). Wieviele Sätze beim Krafttraining? Theorie und Praxis [How much sets in strength training? Theory and practice]. *Leistungssport, 28*(3), 50-51.

Kraemer, W. J. (1997). A series of studies - the physiological basis for strength training in American football: fact over philosophy. *Journal of Strength and Conditioning Research, 11*(3), 131-142.

Kraemer, W. J. (2002). Developing a strength training workout. In W. J. Kraemer & K. Häkkinen (Eds.), *Strength training for sport* (pp. 37-54). Oxford: Blackwell Science.

Kraemer, W. J., Ratamess, N., Fry, A. C., Triplett-McBride, T., Koziris, L. P., Bauer, J. A., et al. (2000). Influence of resistance training volume and periodization on physiological and performance adaptations in collegiate women tennis players. *The American Journal of Sports Medicine, 28*(5), 626-633.

Kramer, J. B., Stone, M. H., O'Bryant, H. S., Conley, M. S., Johnson, R. L., Nieman, D. C., et al. (1997). Effects of single vs. multiple sets of weight training: impact of volume, intensity, and variation. *Journal of Strength and Conditioning Research, 11*(3), 143-147.

Leighton, J. R., Holmes, D., Benson, J., Wooten, B., & Schmerer, R. (1967). A study on the effectiveness of ten different methods of progressive resistance exercise on the development of strength, flexibility, girth and bodyweight. *Journal of the Association of Physical and Mental Rehabilitation, 21*(3), 78-81.

Marées, H. de (2002). *Sportphysiologie [Physiology of sports]* (9th ed.). Köln: Sport und Buch Strauss.

Martin, D., Carl, K., & Lehnertz, K. (1993). *Handbuch Trainingslehre [Handbook training science]* (2nd ed.). Schorndorf: Hofmann.

Marx, J. O., Ratamess, N. A., Nindl, B. C., Gotshalk, L. A., Volek, J. S., Dohi, K., et al. (2001). Low-volume circuit versus high-volume periodized resistance training in women. *Medicine & Science in Sports & Exercise, 33*(4), 635-643.

McBride, J. M., Triplett-McBride, T., Davie, A., & Newton, R. U. (2002). The effect of heavy- vs. light-load jump squats on the development of strength, power, and speed. *Journal of Strength and Conditioning Research, 16*(1), 75-82.

Mentzer, M. (1996). On overtraining. *Muscular Development, 2*, 46-47, 184.

Messier, S. P., & Dill, M. E. (1985). Alterations in strength and maximal oxygen uptake consequent to Nautilus circuit weight training. *Research Quarterly for Exercise and Sport, 56*(4), 345-351.

Morrissey, M. C., Harman, E. A., Frykman, P. N., & Han, K. H. (1998). Early phase differential effects of slow and fast barbell squat training. *The American Journal of Sports Medicine, 26*(2), 221-230.

Moss, B. M., Refsnes, P. E., Abildgaard, A., Nicolaysen, K., & Jensen, J. (1997). Effects of maximal effort strength training with different loads on dynamic strength, cross-sectional area, load-power and load-velocity relationships. *European Journal of Applied Physiology, 75*(3), 193-199.

Müller, A. (2003). Zur Transferierbarkeit trainingsmethodischer Erfahrungen des Hochleistungsbodybuildings. Eine kritische Betrachtung des vorliegenden Methodenspektrums [Transferability of methodical knowledge by competitive bodybuilding. A critical reflection of currently methods]. *Leistungssport, 33*(4), 38-42.

Ostrowski, K. J., Wilson, G. J., Weatherby, R., Murphy, P. W., & Lyttle, A. D. (1997). The effect of weight training volume on hormonal output and muscular size and function. *Journal of Strength and Conditioning Research, 11*(3), 148-154.

Paulsen, G., Myklestad, D., & Raastad, T. (2003). The influence of volume of exercise on early adaptations to strength training. *Journal of Strength and Conditioning Research, 17*(1), 115-120.

Pereira, M. I. R., & Gomes, P. S. C. (2003). Muscular strength and endurance tests: reliability and prediction of the repetition maximum - Review and new evidences. *Revista Brasileira de Medicina do Esporte, 9*(5), 336-346.

Peterson, M. D., Rhea, M. R., & Alvar, B. A. (2004). Maximizing strength development in athletes: a meta-analysis to determine the dose-response relationship. *Journal of Strength and Conditioning Research, 18*(2), 377-382.

Philipp, M. (1999). Einsatz-Training versus Mehrsatz-Training. Zur Kontroverse um die Satzzahl beim Krafttraining unter Berücksichtigung empirischer Evidenzen [Single-set versus multiple-set training. To adress the controversy under consideration of empirical data]. *Leistungssport, 29*(4), 27-34.

Pollock, M. L. (1998). Muscular hypertrophy responses to 6 months of high- or low-volume resistance training. *Medicine & Science in Sports & Exercise, 30*(5), S116.

Pollock, M. L., Graves, J. E., Bamman, M. M., Legett, S. H., Carpenter, D. M., Carr, C., et al. (1993). Frequency and volume of resistance training: effect on cervical extension strenght. *Archives of Physical Medicine and Rehabilitation, 74*, 1080-1086.

Reid, C. M., Yeather, R. A., & Ullrich, I. H. (1987). Weight training and strength, cardiorespiratory functioning and body composition of men. *British Journal of Sports Medicine, 21*(1), 40-44.

Remmert, H., Schischek, A., Zamhöfer, T., & Ferrauti, A. (2005). Zum Einfluss der Regenerationsdauer auf die Kraft- und Muskelmassenzunahme im Rahmen eines Einsatz-Hochintensitätstrainings (High Intensity Training) [Influence of regeneration period on strength and lean body mass increases in single-set high-intensity training]. *Leistungssport, 35*(2), 15-19.

Rhea, M. R., Alvar, B. A., Ball, S. D., & Burkett, L. N. (2002). Three sets of weight training superior to 1 set with equal intensity for eliciting strength. *Journal of Strength and Conditioning Research, 16*(4), 525-529.

Rhea, M. R., Alvar, B. A., Burkett, L. N., & Ball, S. D. (2003). A meta-analysis to determine the dose response for strength development. *Medicine & Science in Sports & Exercise, 35*(3), 456-464.

Sanborn, K., Boros, R., Hruby, J., Schilling, B., O´Bryant, H. S., Johnson, R. L., et al. (2000). Short-Term Performance Effects of Weight Training With Multiple Sets Not to Failure vs. a Single Set to Failure in Women. *Journal of Strength and Conditioning Research, 14*(3), 328-331.

Schlumberger, A. (2000). *Optimierung von Trainingsstrategien im Schnellkrafttraining [Improvement of power training strategies].* Köln: Sport und Buch Strauß.

Schlumberger, A., & Schmidtbleicher, D. (1999). Einsatz-Training als trainingsmethodische Alternative - Möglichkeiten und Grenzen [Single-set training as methodical alternative - potentials and limits]. *Leistungssport, 29*(3), 9-11.

Schlumberger, A., & Schmidtbleicher, D. (2001). Effekte eines Krafttrainings mit explosiv-isometrischen Kontraktionen [Effects of strength training using fast isometric contractions]. *Deutsche Zeitschrift für Sportmedizin, 52*(3), 94-99.

Schlumberger, A., Stec, J., & Schmidtbleicher, D. (2001). Single- vs. multiple-set strength training in women. *Journal of Strength and Conditioning Research, 15*(3), 284-289.

Schlumberger, A., Wirth, K., Liu, Y., Steinacker, J., & Schmidtbleicher, D. (2003). Effekte eines Trainings mit einer Schnellkrafttrainingsmethodenkombination [Training effects of combined power training methods]. *Leistungssport, 33*(4), 14-18.

Schmidtbleicher, D. (1980). *Maximalkraft und Bewegungsschnelligkeit [Maximum strength and movement velocity].* Bad Homburg: Limpert.

Silvester, L. J., Stiggins, C., McGown, C., & Bryce, G. B. (1981). The effect of variable resistance and free-weight training programs on strength and vertical jump. *National Strength Coaches Association Journal, 3*(6), 30-33.

Starkey, D. B., Pollock, M. L., Ishida, Y., Welsch, M. A., Brechue, W. F., Graves, J. E., et al. (1996). Effect of resistance training volume on strength and muscle thickness. *Medicine & Science in Sports & Exercise, 28*(10), 1311-1320.

Stone, M. H., Johnson, R. L., & Carter, D. R. (1979). A short term comparison of two different methods of resistance training on leg strength and power. *Athletic Training, 14*, 158-160.

Stowers, T., McMillan, J., Scala, D., Davis, V., Wilson, D., & Stone, M. (1983). The short-term effects of three different strength-power training methods. *National Strength and Conditioning Journal, 5*(3), 24-27.

Tan, B. (1999). Manipulating resistance training program variables to optimize maximum strength in men: a review. *Journal of Strength and Conditioning Research, 13*(3), 289-304.

Tidow, G. (1999). Zur Dimensionalität des Adaptationsraums im Bereich von Kraftbeanspruchungen [Dimensions of strength adaptations]. In S. Radandt, R. Grieshaber & W. Schneider (Eds.), *Prävention von arbeitsbedingten Gesundheitsgefahren und Erkrankungen [Prevention of work related illness]* (pp. 41-80). Leipzig: monade Verlag.

Tidow, G., & Wiemann, K. (1993). Zur Interpretation und Veränderbarkeit von Kraft-Zeit-Kurven bei explosiv-ballistischen Krafteinsätzen [Interpretation and variability of strength-time curves of explosiv-balistic strength exertion]. In H. F. Voigt (Ed.), *Bewegungen lesen und antworten [Reading and answering movements]* (pp. 153-192). Ahrensburg: Czwalina.

Toji, H., Suei, K., & Kaneko, M. (1997). Effects of combined training loads on relations among force, velocity, and power development. *Canadian Journal of Applied Physiology, 22*(4), 328-336.

Weineck, J. (2000). *Optimales Training [Optimal training]* (11th ed.). Balingen: PERIMED-spitta.

Westcott, W. L. (1995). *Strength fitness: physiological principles and training techniques* (4th ed.). Madison: Brown & Benchmark.

Westcott, W. L., Winett, R. A., Anderson, E. S., Wojcik, J. R., Loud, R. L., Cleggett, E., et al. (2001). Effects of regular and slow speed resistance training on muscle strength. *Journal of Sports Medicine and Physical Fitness, 41*(2), 154-158.

Wilmore, J. H., & Costill, D. L. (2004). *Physiology of sport and exercise* (3rd ed.). Champaign, IL: Human Kinetics.

Wilson, G. J., Newton, R. U., Murphy, A. J., & Humphries, B. J. (1993). The optimal training load for the development of dynamic athletic performance. *Medicine & Science in Sports & Exercise, 25*(11), 1279-1286.

Winett, R. A. (2004). Meta-analyses do not support performance of multiple sets or high volume resistance training. *Journal of Exercise Physiology online, 7*(5), 10-20.

Wolfe, B. L., LeMura, L. M., & Cole, P. J. (2004). Quantitative analysis of single- vs. multiple-set programs in resistance training. *Journal of Strength and Conditioning Research, 18*(1), 35-47.

Zatsiorsky, V. M. (1996). *Krafttraining - Wissenschaft und Praxis [Science and practice of strength training]*. Aachen: Meyer & Meyer.

JÜRGEN GIEßING

The concept of the hypothetical maximum (h1-RM) as a safe alternative to maximum single repetitions

Keywords: hypothetical maxmimum, repetition, intensity, predicting, 1-RM

Introduction

It is generally accepted that muscular hypertrophy is best achieved by realising the maximum number of repetitions in a set (Bührle & Werner, 1984; Tesch & Larsson, 1982; Zatsiorsky, 1996). Those repetitions are called repetition maximums (DeLorme & Watkins, 1951) and the letters RM are added to the number of repetitions. The term "intensity" needs to be dealt with in detail since it is used to describe two different things: It describes the relative amount of weight which is used for a certain exercise and it describes how much effort is being put into doing the exercise. Training for muscular hypertrophy requires submaximal weights but maximal effort. This means that a weight which can be lifted six times but not seven times, represents an athlet´s 6-RM. In order to calculate the relative intensity of that lift it is essential to know his or her 1-RM for this particular exercise.

Single maximum tests (1-RM tests)

According to the advice given in the literature, design and evaluation of resistance training programs are usually based on 1-RM tests. They are used in order to find out the current maximal lifting capacity. According to Ehlenz, Grosser and Zimmermann (2003) 1-RM tests are necessary in order to determine the current strength level of an athlete. Grosser, Brüggemann and Zintl (1986) agree with this concept and base the planning of resistance training programs on the initial 1-RM tests. Schmidtbleicher (1985) points out that 1-repetition-maximum (1-RM) tests should be used on a regular basis in order to evaluate if the current training program still produces improvements in strength. Grosser et al. (1986) agree with this argument and recommend 1-RM tests after each macrocycle in order to adjust the resistances used in the training program to the improved strength levels. However, despite of all these advantages of 1-RM tests, several authors point out that there are several conditions under which single maximum lifts should be avoided. According to Buskies and Boeckh-Behrens (1999) single maximum lifts should not be tried by inexperienced athletes or those with existing internal or orthopaedic problems.

In addition to this, it should also be taken into consideration that 1-RM tests may be fairly accurate in order to determine the 1-RM but cannot be considered to be flawless. Before 1-RM testing can take place athletes must warm up properly in order to avoid injury and then find out their 1-RM by a series of maximum lifts. The warming up may already result in some kind of fatigue, even if adequate rest is assured between warm-up sets. If 1-RM testing is being conducted by inexperienced athletes it is particularly difficult, especially if there are no former test results for that athlete. In this cases testing involves a lot of guesswork. Then a weight has to be chosen which might represent the athlete's 1-RM. After this the athlete either completes a full repetition with that weight or fails to complete a full repetition. Choosing a weight which is too heavy increases the risk of injury and in addition to that, the effort put into the failed repetition may also contribute to fatigue. Then the weight has to be decreased and the athlete has to try again and so on. This procedure in combination with the necessity of an adequate warm-up increases the risk of the results may not being as reliable due to the fatigue that is caused by such a testing procedure. Morales and Sobonya (1996) recommend the following testing procedure for 1-RM tests. If there are results of former 1-RM tests then these are used to calculate the percentages of 1-RM for the warm up sets. If the athlete does not know his own 1-RM, then the weights are estimated:

1. 1 set light warm-up (60 % of previous or estimated 1-RM) for ten reps,
2. 1 set moderate warm-up (70 % of previous or estimated 1-RM) for 8 reps,
3. 1 set moderate warm-up (80 % of previous or estimated 1-RM) for 4 reps,
4. 1 set moderate warm-up (85 % of previous or estimated 1-RM) for 2 reps,
5. 1 to 5 sets of 1-RM until the maximum value was reached.

This means that "the" 1-RM test actually consists of a whole series of sets. In order to test the 1-RM by single maximum lifts five to nine sets of 25 to 30 very intense repetitions are necessary which makes it very obvious why some authors doubt the accuracy of single maximum lifts because they believe that the fatigue which is induced by such an intense testing procedure may prevent the individual from attaining a true maximum (Welday, 1988). Another problem is that this testing procedure is based on the results of former tests or even on estimated strength levels. Furthermore it could be shown by Ploutz-Snyder and Giamis (2001) that it takes at least three to four testing sessions to achieve reliable results. Older subjects who were unfamiliar with strength training needed at least eight testing sessions. Because of these problems several authors have tried to develop alternative ways of determining the 1-RM. In 1984 Landers published a table called "maximum based on reps" based on the assumption that one maximum repetition represents 100 %, two reps represent 95 %, four reps 90 %, six reps 85 %, eight reps represent 80 % and ten reps represent 75 % of the maximum.

Table 1: Maximum (pounds) based on reps (Landers, 1984)

1-RM	2-RM	4-RM	6-RM	8-RM	10-RM
400.00	380.00	360.00	340.00	320.00	300.00
395.00	375.25	355.50	335.75	316.00	296.25
390.00	370.50	351.00	331.50	312.00	292.50
385.00	365.75	346.50	327.25	308.00	288.75
380.00	361.00	342.00	323.00	304.00	285.00
375.00	356.25	337.50	318.75	300.00	281.25
370.00	351.50	333.00	314.50	296.00	277.50
365.00	346.75	328.50	310.25	292.00	273.75
360.00	342.00	324.00	306.00	288.00	270.00
355.00	337.25	319.50	301.75	284.00	266.25
350.00	332.50	315.00	279.50	280.00	262.50
345.00	327.75	310.50	293.25	276.00	258.75
340.00	323.00	306.00	289.00	272.00	255.00
335.00	318.25	301.50	284.75	268.00	251.25
330.00	313.50	297.50	280.50	264.00	247.50
325.00	308.75	292.50	276.25	260.00	243.75
320.00	304.00	288.00	272.00	256.00	240.00
315.00	299.25	283.50	267.75	252.00	236.25
310.00	294.50	279.00	263.50	248.00	232.75
305.00	289.75	274.50	259.25	244.00	228.75
300.00	285.00	270.00	255.00	240.00	225.00
295.00	280.25	265.50	250.75	236.00	221.25
290.00	275.50	261.00	246.50	232.00	217.50
285.00	270.75	256.50	242.25	228.00	213.75
280.00	266.00	252.00	238.00	224.00	210.00
270.00	256.50	243.00	229.50	216.00	202.50
265.00	251.75	238.50	225.25	212.00	198.75
260.00	247.00	234.00	221.00	208.00	195.00
255.00	242.25	229.50	216.75	204.00	191.25
250.00	237.50	225.00	212.50	200.00	187.50

Percentages for odd numbers of repetitions or for repetitions higher than ten are not given. A similar correlation between repetitions and percentages of 1-RM was published by Poliquin (1987) who gave an overview of repetitions between 1-RM and 20-RM and their corresponding percentages of 1-RM (cf. table 2).

Table 2: Percentages of maximum and repetition maximums (Poliquin, 1987)

percent of maximum	maximum number of repetitions
60.6	20
61.6	19
62.7	18
63.9	17
65.0	16
66.2	15
67.5	14
68.8	13
70.3	12
72.3	11
74.4	10
76.5	9
78.8	8
80.7	7
83.1	6
85.6	5
88.1	4
90.6	3
94.3	2
100.0	1

Several studies have been conducted in order to evaluate the reliability of the data presented by Landers (Hoeger, Baratte, Hale, & Hopkins, 1987, 1990; Morales & Sobonya, 1996). Those studies found the data published by Landers to be helpful for some exercises whereas they were not found to be useful for all exercises:

> "The data indicates that the number of repetitions performed at selected percentages of the 1-RM is not the same for all lifts (...). For example, when working at 60 percent of the 1-RM, 33.9 repetitions on the leg press were performed on average, while on the arm curl only 15.3 could be performed."(Hoeger et al., 1987, p. 13)

A high correlation, however, was found for all exercises that involve a relatively large amount of muscle mass (Hoeger et al., 1987, p. 13). In the meantime, several authors have developed formulas which make it possible to calculate the weight that can be lifted for a single maximum repetition (table 3).

Table 3: Formulas for predicting 1-RM from submaximal strength tests

formula	source
% 1-RM = 102.78-2.78 x reps	Brzycki (1993, pp. 88-90)
% 1-RM = 101.3-2.67123 x reps	Landers (1984, p. 60)
% 1-RM = 52.2+41.9 und –0.055 x reps	Mayhew, Ball, Arnold and Bowen (1992, pp. 200-206)
% 1-RM = (0.033 x reps) x resistance + resistance	Epley (1985)
% 1-RM = resistance x (reps $^{0.1}$)	Lombardi (1998, p. 201)
% 1-RM = 0.025 (resistance x reps) + resistance	O'Conner, Simmons and O´Shea (1998, pp. 26-33)

The reliability of these formulas has been measured in several studies (Mayhew, Clemens et al., 1995). When ten or fewer repetitions were used for the submaximal test the most reliable results were found when the following formula was used: % of 1-RM = 102.78 – 2.78 x repetitions.

The hypothetical maximum (h1-RM)

Based on the formula: % of 1-RM = 102.78 – 2.78 x repetitions, the concept of the hypothetical maximum (h1-RM) was developed (Gießing, 2002, 2003). First of all, the formula was transferred into a table that shows how many repetitions can be done at certain percentages of 1-RM (cf. table 4).

Table 4: The h1-RM based on the formula by Brzycki (cf. Gießing, 2003)

percent of maximum	maximum number of repetitions
47.18	20
49.96	19
52.74	18
55.52	17
58.30	16
61.08	15
63.86	14
66.64	13
69.42	12
72.20	11
74.98	10
77.76	9
80.54	8
83.32	7
86.10	6
88.10	5
91.66	4
94.44	3
97.22	2
100.0	1

Using the concept of the h1-RM is a reliable method to predict the 1-RM from submaximal tests. Calculating the h1-RM based on the formula mentioned above is a reliable way to plan and evaluate resistance training programs for athletes who cannot do single maximum repetitions. According to LeSuer, McCormick, Mayhew, Wasserstein and Arnold (1997) the accuracy of predicting the h1-RM from this formula was very high (between 0.96 and 0.99 for the basic compound exercises). These findings are very important because they show that the concept of the hypothetical maximum (h1-RM) may indeed be suitable for designing resistance training programs although predicting the 1-RM from submaximal tests is a method that has been criticized by several authors. Buskies and Boeckh-Behrens (1999, p. 4) compared several older formulas for predicting the 1-RM (cf. Hartmann & Tünnemann, 1993; Riekert, 1993; Starischka, 1995) and found inconsistent conclusions. Intensities which allowed for five repetitions according to one author were supposed to allow for as much as ten to twelve repetitions according to other authors. This inconsistency is also criticized by Marschall and Fröhlich (1999) and Fröhlich, Schmidtbleicher and Emrich (2002).

One aspect all authors agree upon is that predicting the 1-RM is a very individual matter. That means the 1-RM can be predicted very reliably from submaximal strength tests for an individual but is not a suitable way for comparing strength levels of different individuals.

Practical application of the h1-RM

The results of recent studies have documented very well that the 1-RM can be predicted from submaximal tests as shown by Mayhew et al. (1995) and LeSuer et al. (1997). Especially for compound exercises like the bench press, the deadlift or the squat correlations between predicted 1-RM and actual 1-RM were greater than 0.95. For the bench press correlations were between 0.98 and 0.99.

There are several ways the concept of the h1-RM can be used in practical training: 1-RM tests are no longer necessary as the basis of planning resistance training programs for beginners. Instead the 1-RM can be predicted from submaximal tests. If an athlete manages to do ten repetitions with 40 kg but fails to complete an eleventh repetition, then this represents his individual 10-RM. According to the concept of the hypothetical 1-RM his h1-RM for this particular exercise would be 74.98 kg.

Now that this person knows his/her h1-RM an individual resistance training program can be designed. If this individual trains for muscular hypertrophy, the intensity should be between 70 % and 85 % (Martin, 1979, p. 14). This means that weights between 37.5 and 45.5 kg should be used for this exercise. During the following weeks, the h1-RM has to be calculated regularly and when it goes up, the weights have to be adjusted accordingly.
Analysing the development of the h1-RM during a training period gives the athlete some feedback as to whether or not he/she is still making progress on a particular exercise. It is still not known how long athletes should rest between two workouts for the same muscle. Studies show that there are huge interindividual differences (Fry et al., 1994).
Callister et al. (1990) suggest determining the 1-RM regularly. By applying the concept of the h1-RM this can be done without potentially jeopardizing the safety of the lifter by doing maximal tests. Since many athletes - especially on a competitive level - use periodised strength training programs, regularly calculating the h1-RM can give the athlete some feedback if progress is still being made and therefore provide important data for finding out the optimal time to switch from one training period to the next. The concept of the h1-RM is a practical alternative for the traditional testing parameters “Total Force” (TF) and “Fatigue Rate” (FR).
Several authors have used the TF to determine the intensity of a training session. The TF is defined as the product of the multiplication of the weight(s) used and the number of repetitions (Sforzo & Touey, 1996). Bench pressing 40 kg for 50 repetitions represents a TF of 2000 kg, as well as 25 repetitions with 80 kg or 100 repetitions with 20 kg or eight repetitions with 250 kg. A closer look at these different lifts which all represent the same TF shows how problematic the TF is as a test criteria. 100 repetitions with 20 kg should not be a problem for most lifters, even for beginners. 25 repetitions with 80 kg are something that not every recreational lifter could do and eight repetitions with 250 kg are impossible even for world-class lifters. If you compare the 1-RMs of the lifts mentioned, this becomes very obvious: 12 repetitions with 160 kg would be a h1-RM of 230.5 kg and eight repetitions with 250 kg would be a h1-RM of 310.4 kg. This example illustrates that using the h1-RM as an indicator of the intensity of a certain set is much more reliable than the Total Force (TF). The same can be said of the Fatigue Rate (FR) which is calculated on the basis of the TF. The FR describes the development of the TF during several sets

of the same exercise. If an athlete does three sets of a certain exercise, a typical scheme could be:

Table 5: Set, repetitions weight, total force and fatigue rate

set	repetitions x weight	total force	fatigue rate
1st set	10 x 60 kg	600 kg	---
2nd set	6 x 60 kg	480 kg	120 kg
3rd set	10 x 50 kg	500 kg	- 20 kg

In this example, the TF of the first set is 600 kg, 480 kg in the second set and 500 kg in the third set. This means that the FR between the first and the second set is 120 kg (600 kg - 480 kg) and -20 kg between the second and the third set. A negative FR would mean that there is no fatigue but in fact an increase in power which is certainly not the case in the example mentioned above which can be demonstrated very well by a comparison of the h1-RMs of the three sets:

Table 6: Set, repetitions weight, h1-RM and fatigue rate

set	repetitions x weight	h1-RM	fatigue rate
1st set	10 x 60 kg	80.0 kg	---
2nd set	6 x 60 kg	74.5 kg	5.5 kg
3rd set	10 x 50 kg	66.7 kg	7.8 kg

If the fatigue rate is calculated based on the h1-RM, results are much more reliable: The FR between the first and the second set is 5.5 kg (80 kg - 74.5 kg) and 7.8 kg between the second and the third set (74.5 kg - 66.7 kg).

Limitations of the concept

In order to use the concept of the h1-RM efficiently, it is mandatory to also be aware of the limitations of this concept:
Predicting the 1-RM from submaximal tests has only been found to be reliable for compound exercises like the squat, the deadlift and bench press but not for single-joint exercises, the so-called "isolation" exercises (Hoeger et al., 1987, 1990). The h1-RM can only be predicted reliably if the submaximal tests are done within the range of 2 - 20 repetitions. Repetitions for submaximal tests should not exceed 20 or results will be less reliable (Arnold, Mayhew, LeSuer, & McCormick, 1995, p. 205-206). Tests for calculating the h1-RM are most reliable when based on submaximal tests of five to ten repetitions (Bryant & Peterson, 1999).

The h1-RM can not be used to compare strength levels of different athletes (Buskies & Boeckh-Behrens, 1999, pp. 4-8; Hoeger et al., 1987, pp. 11-13). The only parameters that should be compared are the different h1-RMs of an athlete for a particular exercise. That means it is possible to analyse whether or not an athlete improves his strength levels for that exercise during a period of training.

Conclusion

The concept of the individual hypothetical maximum (h1-RM) is not intended to replace the traditional testing procedures but can serve as a suitable alternative, especially if single repetition maximum tests are to be avoided for one reason or another. In these cases the h1-RM can be used very efficiently for predicting an athlete's 1-RM as the foundation of designing resistance training programs for beginners. Predicting the h1-RM may also provide important information about the progress of an athlete's current training program. In addition to this, calculating the FR based on the h1-RM seems to provide more reliable results compared to using TF.

References

Arnold, M. D., Mayhew, J. L., LeSuer, D., & McCormick, M. (1995). Accuracy of predicting bench press and squat performance from repetitions at low and high intensity. *Journal of Strength and Conditioning Research, 9*(9), 205-206.

Bryant, C. X., & Peterson, J. A. (1999). *Measuring strength*, from http://www.fitnessworld.com/library/measure695.html

Brzycki, M. (1993). Strength testing - Predicting a one-rep max from reps-to-fatigue. *Journal of Physical Education, Recreation & Dance, 64*, 88-90.

Bührle, M., & Werner, E. (1984). Das Muskelquerschnittstraining der Bodybuilder [Muscle-hypertrophy training by bodybuilders]. *Leistungssport, 14*(3), 5-9.

Buskies, W., & Boeckh-Behrens, W.-U. (1999). Probleme bei der Steuerung der Trainingsintensität im Krafttraining auf der Basis von Maximalkrafttests [Problems concerning the management of training intensity in strength training]. *Leistungssport, 29*(3), 4-8.

Callister, R., Callister, R. J., Fleck, S. J., & Dudley, G. A. (1990). Physiological and performance responses to overtraining in elite judo athletes. *Medicine & Science in Sports & Exercise, 22*(6), 816-824.

DeLorme, T., & Watkins, A. L. (1951). *Progressive resistance exercise*. New York: Appleton-Cebturs-Croft.

Ehlenz, H., Grosser, M., & Zimmermann, E. (2003). *Krafttraining. Grundlagen, Methoden, Übungen, Leistungssteuerung, Trainingsprogramme [Strength training. Basics, methods, exercises, performance management, training programs]* (7th ed.). München: BLV Verlagsgesellschaft mbH.

Epley, B. (1985). *Poundage chart. Boyd Epley workout*. Lincoln, Nebrasca.

Fröhlich, M., Schmidtbleicher, D., & Emrich, E. (2002). Belastungssteuerung im Muskelaufbautraining. Belastungsnormativ Intensität versus Wiederholungszahl [Training control in hypertrophy training. Intensity vs. repetition]. *Deutsche Zeitschrift für Sportmedizin, 53*(3), 79-83.

Fry, A. C., Kraemer, W. J., Van Borselen, F., Lynch, J. M., Marsit, J. L., Roy, E., et al. (1994). Performance decrements with high-intensity resistance exercise overtraining. *Medicine & Science in Sports & Exercise, 26*(9), 1165-1173.

Gießing, J. (2002). *Das Muskelaufbautraining der Bodybuilder. Eine kritische Analyse aus sportwissenschaftlicher Sicht [The hypertrophy training complex used in bodybuilding - a critical analysis from a sport scientific perspective]*. Marburg: Tectum Verlag.

Gießing, J. (2003). Trainingsplanung und -steuerung beim Muskelaufbautraining. Das Konzept vom individuellen hypothetischen Maximalgewicht (h1-RM) als methodische Alternative [Planning and management of training for muscle hypertrophy training. The concept of the individual hypothetical maximum (h1-RM) as a methodological alternative]. *Leistungssport, 33*(4), 26-31.

Grosser, M., Brüggemann, P., & Zintl, F. (1986). *Leistungssteuerung in Training und Wettkampf [Performance management for training and competition]*. München: BLV.

Hartmann, J., & Tünnemann, H. (1993). *Modernes Krafttraining [Modern strength training]*. Berlin: Ullstein.

Hoeger, W., Baratte, S., Hale, D., & Hopkins, D. (1987). Relationship between repetitions and selected percentages of one repetition maximum. *Journal of Applied Sport Science Research, 1*(1), 11-13.

Hoeger, W., Baratte, S., Hale, D., & Hopkins, D. (1990). Relationship between repetitions and selected percentages of one repetition maximum: A comparison between untrained and trained males and females. *Journal of Applied Sport Science Research, 4*(2), 47-54.

Landers, J. (1984). Maximum based on reps. *National Strength and Conditioning Association Journal, 6*(6), 60-61.

LeSuer, D. A., McCormick, J. H., Mayhew, J. L., Wasserstein, R. L., & Arnold, M. D. (1997). The accuracy of prediction equations for estimating 1-RM performance in the bench press, squat, and deadlift. *Journal of Strength and Conditioning Research, 11*(4), 211-213.

Lombardi, V. P. (1989). *Beginning weight training*. Dubuque, IA: Brown.

Marschall, F., & Fröhlich, M. (1999). Überprüfung des Zusammenhangs von Maximalkraft und maximaler Wiederholungszahl bei deduzierten submaximalen Intensitäten [Testing the correlation between maximal strength and repetition maximum for deduced lower levels of intensity]. *Deutsche Zeitschrift für Sportmedizin, 50*(10), 311-315.

Martin, D. (1979). *Grundlagen der Trainingslehre [Fundamentals of training theory]*. Schorndorf: Hofmann.

Mayhew, J. L., Ball, T. E., Busby, K. L., Arnold, M. D., & Bowen, J. C. (1992). Relative muscular endurance performance as a predictor of bench press strength in college men and women. *Journal of Applied Sport Science Research, 6*, 200-206.

Mayhew, J. L., Clemens, J. C., Busky, K. L., Cannon, J. S., Ware, J. S., & Brown, J. C. (1995). Cross-validation of equations to predict 1-RM bench press from repetitions-to-failure. *Medicine & Science in Sports & Exercise, 27*, S209.

Mayhew, J. L., Prinster, J. L., Ware, J. S., Zimmer, D. L., Arabas, J. R., & Bemben, M. G. (1995). Muscular endurance repetitions to predict bench press strength in men of different training levels. *Journal of Sports Medicine and Physical Fitness, 35*(2), 108-113.

Mentzer, M. (1996). On overtraining. *Muscular Development, 2*, 46-47, 184.

Morales, J., & Sobonya, S. (1996). Use of submaximal repetition tests for predicting 1-RM strength in class athletes. *Journal of Strength and Conditioning Research, 10*(3), 186-189.

O´Conner, B., Simmons, J., & O´Shea, P. (1998). *Weigth Training Today*. St Paul:West Publ.

Ploutz-Snyder, L. L., & Giamis, E. L. (2001). Orientation and familiarization to 1-RM strength testing in old and young women. *Journal of Strength and Conditioning Research, 15*(4), 519-523.

Poliquin, C. (1987). *Strength training for elite athletes*. Las Vegas: ASCA-World Clinic Yearbook.

Riekert, H. (1993). Krafttraining im Breitensport [Strength training in recreational sport]. *Deutsche Zeitschrift für Sportmedizin, 44*(7), 312.

Schmidtbleicher, D. (1985). Diagnose des Maximal- und Schnellkraftverhaltens [Diagnosis of maximum strength and power development]. In M. Bührle (Ed.), *Grundlagen des Maximal- und Schnellkrafttrainings [Fundamentals of maximum strength and power training]*. Schorndorf: Hofmann.

Sforzo, G. A., & Touey, P. R. (1996). Manipulating exercise order affects muscular performance during a resistance exercise training session. *Journal of Strength and Conditioning Research, 10*(1), 20-24.

Starischka, S. (1995). *Fit und Gesund [Fit and healthy]*. Niederhausen: Falken Verlag.

Tesch, P. A., & Larsson, L. (1982). Muscle hypertrophy in bodybuilders. *European Journal of Applied Physiology and Occupational Physiology, 49*(3), 301-306.

Welday, J. (1988). Should you check for strength with periodic lifts? *Scholastic Choach, 57*, 49-68.

Zatsiorsky, V. M. (1996). *Krafttraining - Wissenschaft und Praxis [Science and practice of strength training]*. Aachen: Meyer & Meyer.

MICHAEL FRÖHLICH, DIETMAR SCHMIDTBLEICHER & EIKE EMRICH

The accuracy of prediction equations for estimating 1-RM performance

Keywords: prediction, equations, 1-RM, strength training, number of repetition

Introduction

Strength tests are used for a variety of populations, from elite athletes to recreational fitness enthusiasts or males and females in leisure sports. The main reasons for performing strength tests are evaluating initial strength levels and assessing changes in strength. The most frequent and best procedure for evaluating strength is the 1-repetition-maximum (1-RM) technique in which the most weight that can be lifted successfully through a full range of motion (ROM) is used (see Fleck & Kraemer, 1997, p. 98). Furthermore, the 1-RM is a main value for estimating training gains as well as predicting the load for different training settings or submaximal exercise performance (cf. Abadie & Wentworth, 2000, p. 2).

Although less injury data are available on the use of the 1-RM technique (Brown, 1998), the potential for orthopedical injury, and cardiovascular disease may be magnified with maximal or near maximal loads (MacDougall, Tuxen, Sale, Moroz, & Sutton, 1985). Kraemer and Dziados (Kraemer & Dziados, 2002, p. 163) have been shown that strength training is one of the safest physical activities and exercises that can be carried out. Paramount to this is the use of proper exercise technique, safe equipment, proper spotting and appropriate supervision. A lot of equations for estimating percent 1-RM or 1-RM have been reported. However, many of these equations were listed differently in the literature. On the one hand, some of this equations were described in the original article as percent of 1-RM (see Bryzcki, 1993; Epley, 1985; Landers, 1984; O´Connor, Simmons, & O´Shea, 1989). On the other hand the same authors describe the equations for predicting 1-RM (see LeSuer, McCormick, Mayhew, Wasserstein, & Arnold, 1997, p. 211). Afterwards, only the equations for predicting 1-RM from repetitions were evaluated. These equations are listed in table 2.

Table 1: Some equations to predict percent 1-RM from repetitions (cf. Mayhew et al., 1995, p. 110)

authors	equations to predict % 1-RM from repetitions
Brzycki (1993)	% 1-RM = 102.78 - 2.78 x Reps
Epley (1985)	% 1-RM = (0.033 x Reps) x Rep Wt + Rep Wt
Landers (1984)	% 1-RM = 101.3 - 2.67123 x Reps
Mayhew, Ball and Arnold (1989)	% 1-RM = 93.2 - 1.84 Reps + 0.023 $Reps^2$
O´Conner et al. (1989)	% 1-RM = 0.025 x (Rep Wt x Reps) + Rep Wt

Table 2: Some equations to predict 1-RM from repetitions (cf. LeSuer et al., 1997, p. 211)

authors	equations to predict 1-RM from repetitions
Abadie, Altorfer and Schuler (1999)	1-RM = 8.841 + (1.1828 x 7-10 RM)
Brzycki (1993)	1-RM = 100 x Rep Wt / (102.78 - 2.78 x reps)
Epley (1985)	1-RM = (1 + 0.0333 x Reps) x rep wt
Kravitz, Akalan, Nowicki, and Kinzey (2003)	1-RM = 90.66 + (0.085 x Reps x RepsWT) + (-5.306 x Reps)
Landers (1984)	1-RM = 100 x rep wt / (101.3 - 2.67123 x reps)
O´Connor et al. (1989)	1-RM = rep wt (1 + 0.025 x reps)

The basis of the formulas is the strong association between 1-RM and the number of repetitions needed to reach fatigue (cf. LeSuer et al., 1997, p. 211). Rose and Ball (1992, p. 106) describe that, absolute endurance (35 or 45 repetitions to failure), plus body weight, was more effective for predicting bench press 1-RM than absolute muscular endurance alone. The equation was: 1-RM (bench press) = (0.571 x R) + (0.142 X BW) + 20.10 [R = number of repetitions using the 20.4 kg barbell; BW = subject´s body weight].

Many of these prediction equations under- or overestimated the 1-RM respectively percent 1-RM (cf. Mayhew et al., 1995, p. 112; Ware, Clemens, Mayhew, & Johnston, 1995, p. 101). On the other hand, another very important concept of progressive resistance training is the specifying by the load which can be lifted a given number of times (10-RM as well). Furthermore a lot of authors showed no fixed ratio between intensity (percent of 1-RM) and the number of repetitions (Bayer & Ramlow, 1993; Buskies & Boeckh-Behrens, 1999; Fröhlich, 2003; Fröhlich & Schmidtbleicher, 2003; Hoeger, Barette, Hale, & Hopkins, 1987; Hoeger, Hopkins, Barette, & Hale, 1990). Hoeger et al. (1990) have indicated that an individual does not performe the same number of repetitions in different exercises using the same relative amount of the 1-RM. It may be that different prediction equations may be needed for different lifts (cf. Morales & Sobonya, 1996). It was demonstrated that the relationship between percentage of 1-RM and the number of repetitions that can be performed varies with the amount of muscle mass needed to perform the exercise, trained and untrained, men and women, complex or simple exercise and so on (see Fleck & Kraemer, 1997, pp. 99).

Dohoney, Chromiak, Lemire, Abadie and Kovacs (2002, pp. 54) describe such aspects in this area by further investigating:

a) the predictive accuracy of regression equations with untrained and technique-trained subjects,
b) differences in various groups of male subjects,
c) differences in male and female performance,
d) the relationship between performances using different types of resistance training equipment and types of strength exercises, and
e) the validity of repetitions-to-fatigue equations for older adults.

Therefore the purpose of this empirical study was to determine the accuracy of prediction equations for estimating 1-RM performance in various groups and different equations of estimating as well as over many sets.

Materials and methods

Subjects

Thirty-nine male subjects (the subjects represented three categories: 13 untrained (UN), 13 elite track and field athletes (AT) (sprints 100 m and 200 m, long jump and pole vault as well as discus, javelin and shot put) and 13 elite wrestlers (WR) (national and international performance)) were tested in study one. Study two included five untrained men and five elite badminton players (international level). Subjects in study three und study four were male untrained students (N = 6) and untrained men (N = 10). Prior to participation in all studies each individual was advised on the procedure and requirements for the studies and than completed and signed an informed consent document. All subjects were healthy and had no injury. The subjects´ structural dimension descriptives are shown in table 3.

Table 3: Subject structural dimension descriptives in the different studies

	participants (N)	age (yrs)	height (cm)	weight (kg)
study 1	UN (N = 13) AT (N = 13) WR (N = 13)	35.4 ± 7.6 26.1 ± 7.6 25.3 ± 10.6	179.5 ± 5.7 183.5 ± 10.0 175.0 ± 8.8	76.3 ± 5.7 84.6 ± 14.7 77.9 ± 16.1
study 2	untrained men/bad. players (N = 10)	28.5 ± 9.1	178.8 ± 7.2	73.8 ± 6.8
study 3	students (N = 6)	31.8 ± 10.3	180.0 ± 5.8	78.6 ± 7.8
study 4	untrained men (N = 10)	31.3 ± 8.6	179.9 ± 4.5	77.8 ± 7.2

Exercises

The exercise used was bench press at a multi-press. Anderson and Kearney (1982, p. 2) described that the bench press was the exercise selected for use in all testing and training procedures. This exercise was chosen because it was familiar to the subjects, easily administered, and has been shown to be a valid and reliable measure of muscular function.
The subjects held the bar at a position slightly wider than the shoulder width. The position was controlled and recorded. All subjects lowered the bar slowly until it touched the chest and returned it to full arms´ length. Subjects were instructed to exhale as they pushed the bar forward until the arms were near full extended. Prior the 1-RM test attempt, the subjects performed 25 warm-up repetitions with 20 percent of body weight with three minute rest interval. After the warm-up repetitions the 1-RM was determined by the procedure of Anderson and Kearney (1982) (Fröhlich, 2003; Kravitz et al., 2003). In most instances only two or three trials were needed to ascertain the 1-RM. At least a three minute rest was taken between trials. In addition the study 1 was published in Fröhlich (2003), study 2 in Fröhlich, Schmidtbleicher and Emrich (2002), study 3 in Fröhlich, Klein, Emrich and Schmidtbleicher (2004) and study 4 in Fröhlich, Klein, Emrich and Schmidtbleicher (2001).

Maximum number of repetitions

For the maximum number of repetitions at 50 % 1-RM (study 4), 60 % 1-RM (study 1 and study 3), and 85 % 1-RM (study 2), each lifter was instructed to perform as many repetitions as possible, to failure, at the percentage selected for a bench press exercise. All subjects had to carry out 6 sets (study 1, 2 and 4) or 10 sets (study 3) with an one (study 1, 3 and 4) or three (study 2) minute rest interval between the sets. A uniform cadence, with no more than 2-second pause between repetitions, was allowed.

Statistical procedure

All data was entered in the STATISTICA 5.1 statistical analysis software program. Mean and standard deviation data was presented for all subject characteristics. Percent and frequency curve was calculated. One way analysis of variance (ANOVA) and Scheffé post hoc testing were used to identify significant differences among the groups. Paired t-tests were used to evaluate the differences between predicted and actual 1-RM scores in each group and the composite sample (cf. Mayhew et al., 1995, p. 110). Two way analysis of variance (ANOVA) with repeated measurements was used to evaluate differences between groups and series. An alpha level less than or equal to 0.05 was required for statistical significance.

Results

1-RM

The 1-RM in the different studies is shown in figure 1. There was a significant difference between the groups [$F_{(5,59)} = 10.2$; $p < 0.05$]. The AT and the WR had a significantly greater 1-RM bench press compared to the other groups (cf. figure 1). The untrained men (UN) in study 1, untrained and elite badminton players in study 2, students (study 3), and the untrained men in study 4, were not significantly different in 1-RM (cf. table 4).

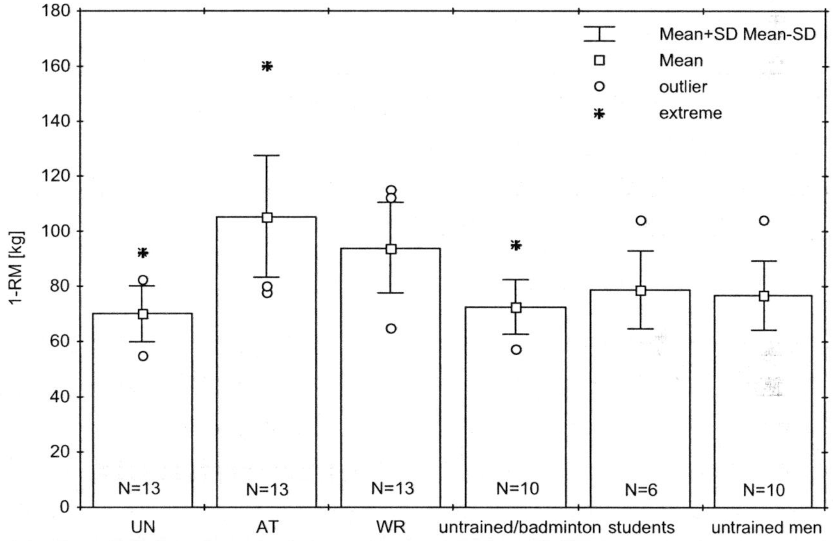

Figure 1: Box-Plot of the 1-RM in the different studies (UN = untrained men, AT = elite track and field athletes, WR = elite wrestlers)

Table 4: p-value of the post hoc Scheffé-Test between the different groups (UN = untrained men, AT = elite track and field athletes, WR = elite wrestlers, untr./bad. = untrained men and badminton players, students = students, untr. men = untrained men)

	UN	AT	WR	untr./bad.	students	untr. men
UN						
AT	p < 0.05					
WR	p < 0.05	p = 0.61				
untr./bad.	p = 1.00	p < 0.05	p = 0.06			
students	p = 0.92	p < 0.05	p = 0.54	p = 0.98		
untr. men	p = 0.95	p < 0.05	p = 0.22	p = 1.00	p = 1.00	

When evaluating the formulas for predicting bench press performance by the equation of Epley (1985) and O´Conner (1989), the predicted 1-RM values did not differ significantly from the achieved 1-RM values. The equation by Brzycki (1993), Kravitz et al. (2003) and Landers (1984) significantly under- or overestimated 1-RM performance, by an average of -48.8 kg to +147.6 kg. Table 5 shows the repetitions, the load, percent 1-RM, achieved 1-RM by the different groups. Table 6 shows the predicted 1-RM in the different groups by the different equations. The equation at higher intensity, for example 85 % 1-RM as well as fewer repetitions, for example 6.3, are better predictors for 1-RM than less intensity and more repetitions (cf. Dohoney et al., 2002). All equations for predicting 1-RM bench press performance can not be used for training control over many sets, because there is no fixed ratio between intensity and repetitions over the sets.

The equation by Epley (1985) [1-RM = (1 + 0.0333 x Reps) x rep wt] and O´Conner et al. (1989) [1-RM = rep wt (1 + 0.025 x reps)] are good predictors for the so-called "hypothetical 1-RM concept" in the first set (cf. Gießing, 2003, 2004). In the further sets, the equations are not usable.

Table 5: Reps, load, percent 1-RM and actual 1-RM by the different groups (mean) (UN = untrained men, AT = elite track and field athletes, WR = elite wrestlers, untr./bad. = untrained men and badminton players, students = students, untr. men = untrained men)

	UN	AT	WR	untr./bad.	students	untr. men
reps	20.6	21.0	22.3	6.3	25.8	30.8
load [kg]	42.0	63.3	56.4	61.6	39.4	38.5
% 1-RM	60 %	60 %	60 %	85 %	50 %	50 %
actual 1-RM	70.0	105.4	94.0	72.5	79.7	76.8

Table 6: Predicted 1-RM in the different groups by different equations (+ sig. different, $p < 0.05$) (UN = untrained men, AT = elite track and field athletes, WR = elite wrestlers, untr./bad. = untrained men and badminton players, students = students, untr. men = untrained men)

equations	UN	AT	WR	untr./bad.	students	untr. men
Brzycki (1993)	92.3+	142.6+	138.3+	72.2	126.9+	224.4+
Epley (1985)	70.8	107.6	98.3	74.5	73.3	78.0
Kravitz et al. (2003)	54.9+	92.2+	79.2+	90.2+	40.2+	28.0+
Landers (1984)	90.7+	140.0+	135.1+	72.9	121.7+	202.4+
O´Conner et al. (1989)	63.6+	96.5	87.8	71.3	64.8	68.2

Repetitions

The repetitions to fatigue at 50 %, 60 % or 85 % 1-RM decreased significantly over the sets in all studies. The highest reduction of the repetitions to fatigue was in the second und third set. The decrease in the further sets (4 to 6 set) was not significantly different. The reduction in the set 4 to 6 showed an individual threshold (cf. figure 2).

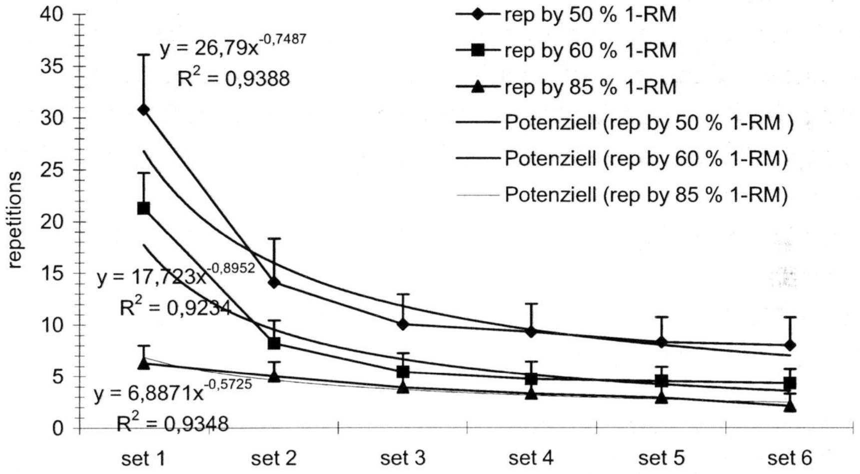

Figure 2: Number of repetitions at 50 % (study 4), 60 % (study 1) and 85 % (study 2) 1-RM over 6 sets as well as potential conformation

The best equations for predicting repetitions over many sets is a potential function (cf. figure 2). The equation at 85 % 1-RM is a better predictor for repetitions, than the equations at 50 % or 60 % 1-RM.

Table 3: Actual und predict repetitions over 6 sets by the potential equation (y = 6.8871x–0.5725) from the value in study 2

	set 1	set 2	set 3	set 4	set 5	set 6
actual reps	6.3	5.0	3.9	3.3	2.9	2.1
predict reps	6.9	4.6	3.7	3.1	2.7	2.5

Discussion and conclusion

Various strength prediction equations have been published including generalized equations and exercise specific equations (cf. Abadie & Wentworth, 2000; Pereira & Gomes, 2003). Some of these equations were described in the original article as percent of 1-RM or as 1-RM. Furthermore, cross-validation studies by Pereira and Gomes (2003, p. 344) showed, that only two of nine equations were validated, for example the study of Mayhew, Ball, Ward, Hart and Arnold (1991) and Epley´s (1985). Additionally, it is possible that specificity has a major influence on the 1-RM relationship, being influenced by the sample, the exercise, the sex and type of performance. Also, prediction equations for estimating 1-RM bench press performance are limited, especially for training control over many sets. Concluding, the predication of 1-RM from submaximal tests (% 1-RM), or even exercise prescription should be carefully considered. Pereira and Gomes (Pereira & Gomes, 2003, p. 344) mention the specificity of the sample (males vs. females, trained vs. untrained), of the exercise (upper limbs vs. lower limbs, multi-joint vs. single joint, big muscle groups vs. small muscle groups), of the age (young vs. old), of the level of strength (very strong vs. less strong).

References

Abadie, B. R., Altorfer, G. L., & Schuler, P. B. (1999). Does a regression equation to predict maximal strength in untrained lifters remain valid when the subjects are technique trained? *Journal of Strength and Conditioning Research, 13*(3), 259-263.

Abadie, B. R., & Wentworth, M. C. (2000). Prediction of one repetition maximum strength from a 5-10 repetition submaximal strength test in college-aged females. *Journal of Exercise Physiology online, 3*(3), 1-6.

Anderson, T., & Kearney, J. T. (1982). Effects of three resistance training programs on muscular strength and absolute and relative endurance. *Research Quarterly for Exercise and Sport, 53*(1), 1-7.

Bayer, G., & Ramlow, J. (1993). Verhältnis von Kraft- und Ausdauerfähigkeit für die Vervollkommnung der Kraftausdauer im Rennrudern [Relationship of strength and endurance skills for strength endurance improvement in rowing sport]. *Leistungssport, 23*(3), 15-19.

Brown, L. E. (1998). Strength testing for children. *Strength and Conditioning Journal, 20*(5), 75.

Brzycki, M. (1993). Strength testing - Predicting a one-rep max from reps-to-fatigue. *Journal of Physical Education, Recreation & Dance, 64*, 88-90.

Buskies, W., & Boeckh-Behrens, W.-U. (1999). Probleme bei der Steuerung der Trainingsintensität im Krafttraining auf der Basis von Maximalkrafttests [Problems concerning the management of training intensity in strength training]. *Leistungssport, 29*(3), 4-8.

Dohoney, P., Chromiak, J. A., Lemire, D., Abadie, B. R., & Kovacs, C. (2002). Prediction of one repetition maximum (1-RM) strength from a 4-6 RM and a 7-10 RM submaximal strength test in healthy young adult males. *Journal of Exercise Physiology online, 5*(3), 54-59.

Epley, B. (1985). *Poundage chart. Boyd Epley workout*. Lincoln, Nebrasca.

Fleck, S. J., & Kraemer, W. J. (1997). *Designing resistance training programs* (2nd ed.). Champaign, IL: Human Kinetics.

Fröhlich, M. (2003). *Kraftausdauertraining. Eine empirische Studie zur Methodik [Strength endurance training. An empirical study]*. Göttingen: Cuvillier.

Fröhlich, M., Klein, M., Emrich, E., & Schmidtbleicher, D. (2001). Arbeit als Bruttokriterium der Belastung im Kraftausdauertraining [Work as gross criterium of the work load in strength endurance training]. *Leistungssport, 31*(2), 24-28.

Fröhlich, M., Klein, M., Emrich, E., & Schmidtbleicher, D. (2004). Belastungsreaktionen beim Kraftausdauertraining (KA-T) über mehrere Serien [Work load responses in strength endurance training (SE-T) on multiple sets]. In H. Riehle (Ed.), *Biomechanik als Anwendungsforschung. Transfer zwischen Theorie und Praxis [Biomechanics in research. Transfer between theory and practice]* (pp. 291-297). Hamburg: Czwalina Verlag.

Fröhlich, M., & Schmidtbleicher, D. (2003). Belastungsintensität und Wiederholungszahl in Abhängigkeit von der Trainingsspezifik im Krafttraining [Dependance of intensity and number of repetitions from training specifity in strength training]. In G.-P. Brüggemann & G. Morey-Klapsing (Eds.), *Biologische Systeme. Mechanische Eigenschaften und ihre Adaptation bei körperlicher Belastung [Biological systems. Mechanical characteristics and adaptations to physical work load]* (pp. 54-58). Hamburg: Czwalina Verlag.

Fröhlich, M., Schmidtbleicher, D., & Emrich, E. (2002). Belastungssteuerung im Muskelaufbautraining. Belastungsnormativ Intensität versus Wiederholungszahl [Training control in hypertrophy training. Intensity vs. repetition]. *Deutsche Zeitschrift für Sportmedizin, 53*(3), 79-83.

Gießing, J. (2003). Trainingsplanung und -steuerung beim Muskelaufbautraining. Das Konzept vom individuellen hypothetischen Maximalgewicht (h1-RM) als methodische Alternative [Planning and management of training for muscle hypertrophy training. The concept of the individual hypothetical maximum (h1-RM) as a methodological alternative]. *Leistungssport, 33*(4), 26-31.

Gießing, J. (2004). *1 Satz Training - Ein wissenschaftlich fundiertes Konzept für schnellstmöglichen Muskelaufbau im Bodybuilding [Single-set training. A concept for rapid muscle gains based on scientific findings]* (1st ed.). Arnsberg: Novagenics.

Hoeger, W. W. K., Barette, S. L., Hale, D. F., & Hopkins, D. R. (1987). Relationship between repetitions and selected percentages of one repetition maximum. *Journal of Applied Sports Science Research, 1*(1), 11-13.

Hoeger, W. W. K., Hopkins, D. R., Barette, S. L., & Hale, D. F. (1990). Relationship between repetitions and selected percentages of one repetition maximum: A comparison between untrained and trained males and females. *Journal of Applied Sport Science Research, 4*(2), 47-54.

Kraemer, W. J., & Dziados, J. (2002). Medical aspects and admininstrative concerns in strength training. In W. J. Kraemer & K. Häkkinen (Eds.), *Handbook of sports medicine and science. Strength training for sport* (pp. 163-175). Oxford: Blackwell Science Ltd.

Kravitz, L., Akalan, C., Nowicki, K., & Kinzey, S. J. (2003). Prediction of 1 repetition maximum in high-school power lifters. *Journal of Strength and Conditioning Research, 17*(1), 167-172.

Landers, J. (1984). Maximum based on reps. *National Strength and Conditioning Association Journal, 6*(6), 60-61.

LeSuer, D. A., McCormick, J. H., Mayhew, J. L., Wasserstein, R. L., & Arnold, M. D. (1997). The accuracy of prediction equations for estimating 1-RM performance in the bench press, squat and deadlift. *Journal of Strength and Conditioning Research, 11*(4), 211-213.

MacDougall, J. D., Tuxen, D., Sale, D. G., Moroz, J. R., & Sutton, J. R. (1985). Arterial blood pressure response to heavy resistance exercise. *Journal of Applied Physiology, 58*(3), 785-790.

Mayhew, J. L., Ball, T. E., & Arnold, M. D. (1989). Prediction of 1-RM bench press from submaximal bench press performance in college males and females. *Journal of Applied Science Research, 3*(3), 73.

Mayhew, J. L., Ball, T. E., Ward, T. E., Hart, C. L., & Arnold, M. D. (1991). Relationship of structural dimensions to bench press strength in college males. *Journal of Sports Medicine and Physical Fitness, 31*(2), 135-141.

Mayhew, J. L., Prinster, J. L., Ware, J. S., Zimmer, D. L., Arabas, J. R., & Bemben, M. G. (1995). Muscular endurance repetitions to predict bench press strength in men of different training levels. *Journal of Sports Medicine and Physical Fitness, 35*(2), 108-113.

Morales, J., & Sobonya, S. (1996). Use of submaximal repetition tests for predicting 1-RM strength in class athletes. *Journal of Strength and Conditioning Research, 10*(3), 186-189.

O´Connor, B., Simmons, J., & O´Shea, P. (1989). *Weight training today*. St. Paul: West Publ.

Pereira, M. I. R., & Gomes, P. S. C. (2003). Muscular strength and endurance tests: reliability and prediction of the repetition maximum - Review and new evidences. *Revista Brasileira de Medicina do Esporte, 9*(5), 336-346.

Rose, K., & Ball, T. E. (1992). A field test for predicting maximum bench press lift of college women. *Journal of Applied Sport Science Research, 6*(2), 103-106.

Ware, J. S., Clemens, C. T., Mayhew, J. L., & Johnston, T. J. (1995). Muscular endurance repetitions to predict bench press squat strength in college football players. *Journal of Strength and Conditioning Research, 9*(2), 99-103.

PETER PREUSS

High-intensity training versus High-volume training

Keywords: Low-volume training, High-volume training, High-intensity training, High-intensity training technique, muscular failure

Introduction

In recent years single-set and multiple-set training aroused again interest in german (Gießing, 2000; Heiduk, Preuss, & Steinhöfer, 2002; Philipp, 1999a, 1999b; Remmert, Schischek, Zamhöfer, & Ferrauti, 2005; Schlumberger & Schmidtbleicher, 1999) and international sport scientific journals (Gießing, 2003; Hass, Garzarella, de Hoyos, & Pollock, 2000; Kemmler, Lauber, Engelke, & Weineck, 2004; Paulsen, Myklestad, & Raastad, 2003; Rhea, Alvar, Ball, & Burkett, 2002; Schlumberger, Stec, & Schmidtbleicher, 2001; Wolfe, Valerio, Strohecker, & Szmedra, 2001). The focus was the training volume necessary to achieve maximum strength increases and hypertrophy adaptations. Meta-analysis (Peterson, Rhea, & Alvar, 2004; Rhea, Alvar, Burkett, & Ball, 2003; Wolfe, LeMura, & Cole, 2004) showed advantages of multiple-set training: "Four sets per muscle group elicited maximal gains in both trained and untrained individuals" (Rhea et al., 2003, p. 456). Apart from methodical flaws (Winett, 2004) there exist various concepts of single-set training with different program variables (Heiduk et al., 2002).

Aim of the study

This study examined the effects of High-intensity training - a special kind of Low-volume training - versus High-volume training (High-volume training as generic term will be used instead of multiple-set training) on maximal strength and body composition. Furthermore the changes observed were set in relation to the program variables "time under tension" and "training volume".
Accordingly to Gießing et al. (2005), High-intensity training (HIT) is defined as 1 to 2 sets per exercise, applying high-intensity training techniques. High-intensity training techniques (HITT) display a special selection of resistance training systems and methods (Fleck & Kraemer, 2004) used in HIT. There are only one or two sets per exercise whereas several exercises might be done for

each muscle group or body region (Weingarten, 2000, p. 321). High-volume training (HVT) is characterized by 2 or more sets per exercise and several exercises per muscle group or body region. Rest intervals between sets are at least 30 seconds. Low-volume training should be done at high intensities of exertion which must be considered to be at least equally effective as high-volume training.

Methods

Six well trained male subjects (age: 25.17 ± 5.42 years, height: 181.83 ± 4.31 cm) with more than six years of strength training experience (3 - 4 training sessions per week) participated in this study. HIT and HVT were originally compared for a period of 8 weeks. Because of fatigue symptoms and motivational problems during the course of HIT this period was reduced to 7 weeks. A transition phase of one week between the two training approaches consisted of 2 to 3 whole body workouts with 2 sets x 10 - 15 repetitions with 50 % training load of HIT (see table 1).

Table 1: Study design

training	week
high-intensity training	0 - 8
pre-test 1	0
training 1	1 - 7
post-test 1	8
transition phase	**9**
high-volume training	10 - 18
pre-test 2	10
training 2	11 - 17
post-test 2	18

Anthropometric measurements included height, body weight, fat mass (FM) and lean body mass (LBM). Body composition was analysed by bioelectric impedance analysis (BIA) using the Tanita body fat analyser scale TBF-532.
1-RM bench press, 3-RM pull-ups as well as isokinetic knee extension and flexion (Cybex 6000) were utilized to measure strength changes.
The study subjects completed both trainings approaches consecutively. The benefit of this procedure is that there is a methodical mix of single case and group analyses which can be used to compare the effectiveness of HIT and HVT (Philipp, 1999b, p. 33). Schlicht (1988, p. 13) is of the opinion that single case studies are particularly advantageous methods for analysing intra-individual performance changes in competitive sport, primarily due to different

individual regeneration and adaptation capacities (see also Harrison, 2000; Johnston, 2000; Kelso, 2000; Szubski, 1999; Weingarten, 2000). The procedure described implies that all observed changes must be interpreted as training adaptations.

Training procedures

The training program was divided in a 3 day split-scheme:

- workout 1: chest, arms,
- workout 2: legs, calves, lower back,
- workout 3: back, shoulders, abdominals.

Each single workout was supervised and documented (training diary). Although many programs are based on training each muscle group twice a week, in this study one to three days were taken off between training sessions to avoid overtraining because of too short regeneration phases, depending on individual regeneration abilities.

A standardized general and specific warm-up was performed before every workout. Training weight was self-selected by study subjects because of training experiences and not calculated as % 1-RM of maximum strength testing. Prescribing an RM is considered to be superior for the following reasons:

1. strength varies about 10 - 20 % over the day,
2. the number of repetitions with a fixed % RM has a wide inter-individual variability and
3. the number of repetitions varies from one muscle to another (Boeckh-Behrens & Buskies, 2000; Tan, 1999).

Researchers also suggested a slightly reduced training load for HIT because of slower repetition speed. For exercise selection two standpoints were considered: on the one hand exercises should effectively stress the particular muscle group (Boeckh-Behrens & Buskies, 2000; Brzycki, 1995), on the other hand study subjects had to be familiar with the exercises to eliminate strength gains through coordinative learning effects. Consequent to the last point three subjects performed following alternative exercises (see table 2):

- squat instead of leg press,
- stiffed-leg deadlift instead of seated leg curl and
- dumbell incline curl instead of machine curl.

Table 2: HIT and HVT programs

	exercises	sets x repetitions	
		HIT	HVT
workout 1	**chest exercises**		
	bench press	1 x 8 - 10 + A/B/A	3 x 8 - 10
	incline press	1 x 8 - 10 + A/B/A	3 x 8 - 10
	machine flies	1 x 8 - 10 + A/Iso/B/A/Iso	3 x 8 - 10
	arm exercises		
	french press	1 x 8 - 10 + A/B/A	3 x 8 - 10
	cable pushdowns	1 x 8 - 10 + A/B/A	3 x 8 - 10
	barbell curl	1 x 8 - 10 + A/B/A	3 x 8 - 10
	machine curl or	1 x 8 - 10 + A/Iso/B/A/Iso	3 x 8 - 10
	dumbell incline curl	1 x 8 - 10 + A/B/A	3 x 8 - 10
workout 2	**leg exercises**		
	leg press or	1 x 10 - 12 + A/B/A	3 x 10 - 12
	squat	1 x 10 - 12 + P/B/P	3 x 10 - 12
	leg extension	1 x 10 - 12 + A/B/A	3 x 10 - 12
	lying leg curl	1 x 10 - 12 + A/Iso/B/A/Iso	3 x 10 - 12
	seated leg curl or	1 x 10 - 12 + A/Iso/B/A/Iso	3 x 10 - 12
	stiffed-leg deadlift	1 x 8 - 10 + B	3 x 8 - 10
	calf exercises		
	bend over calf raise	1 x 10 - 12 + P/B/P/B/P	3 x 10 - 12
	seated calf raise	1 x 8 - 10 + P/B/P	3 x 8 - 10
	lower back		
	back extension	1 x 10 - 12 + Iso/B/Iso	3 x 10 - 12
workout 3	**back exercises**		
	pull-ups	1 x 8-10 + A/Iso/B/A/Iso	3 x 8 - 10
	bent over barbell row	1 x 8-10 + P/B/P	3 x 8 - 10
	dumbell row	1 x 8-10 + A/B/A	3 x 8 - 10
	shoulder exercises		
	dumbell shoulder press	1 x 8 - 10 + A/B/A	3 x 8 - 10
	cable side raise	1 x 8 - 10 + A/B/A	3 x 8 - 10
	core exercises		
	pelvis lift	1 x max.	3 x submax.
	crunches	1 x max.	3 x submax.
	side bridge	1 x max.	3 x submax.

A = assisted positive repetition, B = breakdown set, Iso = isometric contraction, max. = maximum repetitions, P = partial repetitions, submax. = submaximal repetitions.

Descripition of HIT

The applied HIT represents a modification of the training method described by Weingarten (2000) and Yates and Wolff (1995). After an exercise specific warm-up only one training set per exercise beyond the point of momentary muscular failure (PMF) was performed, utilising so called high-intensity training techniques (assisted positive repetitions, breakdown sets, isometric contractions and partial repetitions). The execution of each repetition occurred in accordance to Brzycki´s (1998) "quality reps", abbreviated R E P S:

"**R**efrain from using momentum during the concentric phase.
Emphasize the mid-range position.
Perform the eccentric phase in a deliberate fashion.
Stimulate your muscles throughout the greatest range of motion."

The concentric phase of each repetition took 1 - 2 seconds whereas the eccentric phase was emphasised and lasted 3 - 4 seconds. An exemplary training set consisted of maximal repetitions until PMF followed by 1 - 2 assisted positive repetitions. Afterwards the weight was immediately reduced by 25 - 30 percent and maximal repetitions were performed with the reduced weight until PMF, again followed by 1 - 2 assisted positive repetitions.

Description of HVT

The HVT program was in accordance with the HIT program but differed in the following aspects. Differences existed in

a) the number of sets (3 sets vs. 1 set),
b) repetition speed (normal vs. 2 seconds concentric, 4 seconds eccentric) and
c) not applying of high-intensity training techniques in the HVT group.

Rest between sets and exercises was 2 to 3 minutes.

Analysis of training parameters

Commonly training volume is calculated by *sets x repetitions x weight* used (Baechle, Earle, & Wathen, 2000, p. 418; Fleck & Kraemer, 2004, p. 7). For example, if 100 kg are used to perform 10 repetitions, training volume is 1000 kg (10 x 100 kg = 1000 kg).

The calculation of training volume equals the amount of physical work done:
$w = m \times g \times s$, at which

w = *work*,
m = *mass*,
g = *gravity and*
s = *range of motion*.

Here body or weight displacement is independent of upright or inclined plane movement. It depends only on gravity of body or weight lifted ($m \times g$) and the range of motion (s). Drawing conclusions from physical work to physiological work, expressed as muscle contraction, is difficult.

> "From a theoretical perspective, doing a repetition slowly but with a high intensity should maximize muscle tension..." (Westcott et al., 2001, p. 155)

The muscle is under a constant high tension and momentum is decreased. Despite of lower physical work, the time under tension (TUT) and therefore ATP-depletion as well as physiological work tends overall to be greater.
In conclusion, the author suggests differentiating training volume as a generic term in physical work (total work) and physiological work (time under tension), as shown in figure 1.

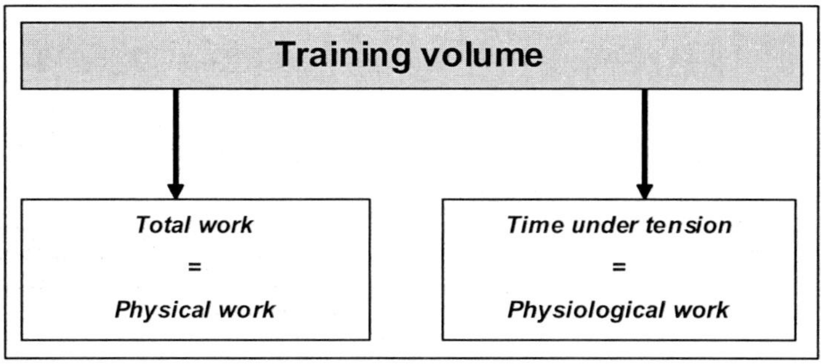

Figure 1: Differentiation of training volume

In this study, time under tension (TUT) and total work (TW) were calculated to compare HIT and HVT. Changes in testing exercises were compared to TUT and TW whereas performance limiting muscle groups for each testing exercise were regarded.

Analysis parameter time under tension (TUT)

In this study the analysis parameter time under tension (TUT) was used as an equivalent to the traditional strength training parameter repetitions (Kieser, 1998). In addition to repetitions the usage of TUT reflects the slower repetition speed in HIT. An equal number of repetitions in HIT causes a longer TUT and thus a higher physiological work. Furthermore high-intensity training techniques (assisted positive repetitions, breakdown sets (also called "drop-sets" or "stripping"), isometric contractions and partial repetitions) will be - in contrast to number of repetitions - included in TUT. In this case calculation of TUT seems to be the more practicable solution.

Table 3 shows TUT per repetition in HIT including high-intensity training techniques. Only the performance limiting muscle groups for each testing exercise were displayed and considered in analysis of training data.

Table 3: Time under tension (TUT) for repetitions including high-intensity training techniques of performance limiting muscle groups for each testing exercise in HIT

test exercise	exercises	execution and TUT [sec.]
knee extension	leg press or	N [6] / I [6] / B [6] / I [6]
	squat	N [6] / I [6] / B [6] / I [6]
	leg extension	N [6] / I [6] / B [6] / I [6]
knee flexion	lying leg curl	N [6] / I [6] / Iso [6] / B [6] / I [6] / Iso [6]
	seated leg curl or	N [5] / I [5] / Iso [6] / B [5] / I [5] / Iso [6]
	stiffed-leg deadlift	N [5] / B [5]
1-RM bench press	bench press	N [5] / I [5] / B [5] / I [5]
	incline press	N [5] / I [5] / B [5] / I [5]
	machine flies	N [5] / I [5] / Iso [6] / B [5] / I [5] / Iso [6]
	french press	N [5] / I [5] / B [5] / I [5]
	cable pushdowns	N [5] / I [5] / B [5] / I [5]
3-RM pull-up	pull-ups	N [5] / I [5] / Iso [6] / B [5] / I [5] / Iso [6]
	bent over barbell row	N [4] / P [2] / B [4] / P [2]
	dumbell row	N [5] / I [4] / B [5] / I [4]
	barbell curl	N [5] / I [5] / B [5] / I [5]
	machine curl or	N [5] / I [5] / B [5] / I [5]
	dumbell incline curl	N [5] / I [5] / B [5] / I [5]
A = assisted positive repetition, B = breakdown set, Iso = isometric contraction, N = normal repetitions, P = partial repetitions, TUT = time under tension.		

Table 4 shows a sample calculation of TUT for pull-ups. Eight regular repetitions to PMF (**N**) were performed using bodyweight and an additional weight of 15 kg followed by two assisted repetitions (**A**). The breakdown set - without any additional weight, only the bodyweight would be lifted - consisted of three repetitions (**B**) to PMF plus one assisted repetition (**A**) and another six seconds lasting isometric contraction (**Iso**). According to the calculation basic of table 3 the total TUT achieved 82 seconds (see table 4).

Table 4: Exemplarily pull-ups calculation of TUT in HIT

repetitions		repetition TUT	TUT
8	N	5 sec.	40 sec.
2	A	5 sec.	10 sec.
1	Iso	6 sec.	6 sec.
3	B	5 sec.	15 sec.
1	A	5 sec.	5 sec.
1	Iso	6 sec.	6 sec.
			82 sec.
A = assisted positive repetition, B = break-down set, Iso = isometric contraction, N = normal repetitions, TUT = time under tension.			

In order to be able to compare the HIT and HVT regimes it is necessary to calculate TUT also for HVT. Exercise-dependend TUT for HVT was fixed between 2 to 4 seconds. For example, three sets of pull-ups at ten, nine and eight repetitions and repetition TUT of 3 seconds led to total TUT of 81 seconds (see table 5).

Table 5: Exemplarily pull-ups calculation of TUT in HVT

repetitions	repetition TUT	TUT
10	3 sec.	30 sec.
9	3 sec.	27 sec.
8	3 sec.	24 sec.
		81 sec.

Analysis parameter total work (TW)

Total work (TW, synonym training volume (Baechle et al., 2000, p. 418; Fleck & Kraemer, 2004, p. 9; Tan, 1999, p. 293)) records the lifted weight over a defined period of time. Generally it is expressed by *number of sets x number of repetitions x lifted weight*. The above mentioned set of pull-ups with a bodyweight of 80 kg and an additional weight of 15 kg resulted in TW of 1270 kg in HIT (see table 6).

Table 6: Exemplarily pull-ups calculation of TW in HIT

repetitions		weight	TW
8	N	95 kg	760 kg
2	A	95 kg	190 kg
3	B	80 kg	240 kg
1	A	80 kg	80 kg
			1270 kg
A = assisted positive repetition, B = breakdown set, N = normal repetitions, TW = total work.			

Isometric contractions were not considered because they represent no physical work. Assisted repetitions were calculated as regular repetitions. Three sets of pull-ups consisting of ten, nine and eight repetitions and a bodyweight of 80 kg plus additional 15 kg led to 2565 kg TW in HVT (see table 7).

Table 7: Exemplarily pull-ups calculation of TW in HVT

repetitions	weight	TW
10	95 kg	950 kg
9	95 kg	855 kg
8	95 kg	760 kg
		2565 kg

Data analysis

Mean and standard deviation data was presented for all subject characteristics. Differences between pre- and post-test and groups were tested with wilcoxon-test (n < 30) or t-test (n > 30), depending on sample size. Testing procedure and p-value is mentioned in the text. Alpha levels less than or equal to 0.05 were required for statistical significance.

Results of all study subjects

Duration of training sessions

Average reduction of time for HIT was significant at 12.46 minutes per session (t-test, p = 0.000). The average duration of overall other activities (other activities are all further athletic activities except strength training, e.g. cycling, running etc.) showed a difference of 11.67 minutes with no statistical significance (wilcoxon-test, p = 0.753).

Table 8: Duration of training sessions and other activities for HIT and HVT in all subjects

	training session [min.]		**other activities [min.]**	
	sum total	mean	sum total	mean
HIT	1418 ± 180.88	72.02 ± 7.31	1094.50 ± 554.12	56.01 ± 10.25
HVT	1774 ± 105.57	84.49 ± 5.03	1082.83 ± 549.62	63.69 ± 6.35
$d_{HIT-HVT}$	-357 ± 257.79	-12.46 ± 7.39*	11.67 ± 424.63	-7.67 ± 13.58
* = significant difference, d = difference; min. = time in minutes				

Anthropometric changes

Wilcoxon-test showed no significant changes in body weight (BW), fat mass (FM) and lean body mass (LBM) for neither HIT nor HVT. As displayed in figure 2 changes in LBM were higher for HIT than HVT. Fat mass (FM) tended to result in advantages in HIT.

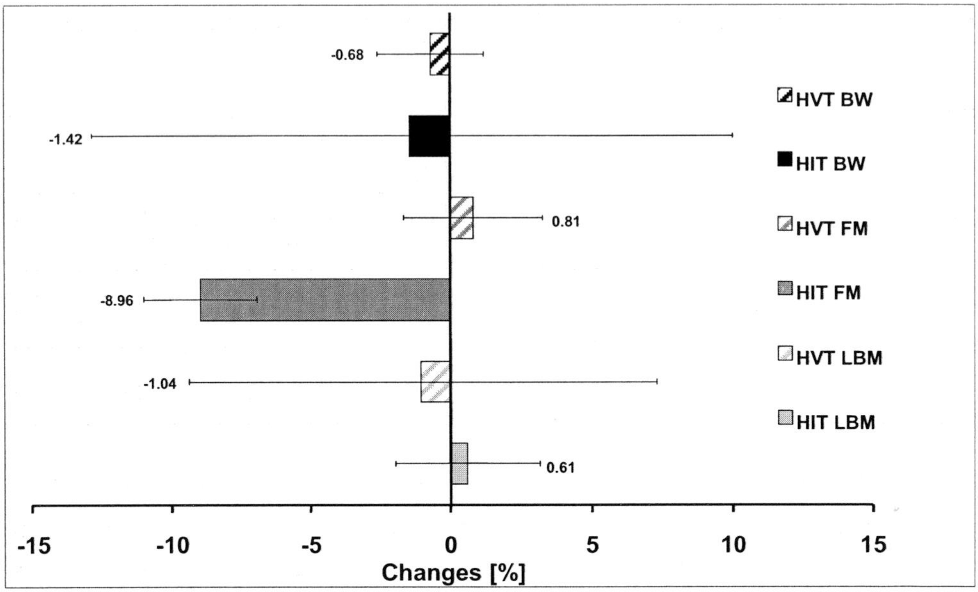

Figure 2: Changes in anthropometric data for HIT and HVT of all subjects (BW = body weight, FM = fat mass, LBM = lean body mass)

Training parameters and test results

Total work (TW) and time under tension (TUT) were calculated. These two parameters could be able to produce muscle hypertrophy and consequently influence the changes between pre- and post-test. Table 9 and 10 show test results for 1-RM bench press and 3-RM pull-ups with no significant differences between HIT and HVT (wilcoxon-test, $p = 0.695$). Training parameters indicated a two times higher TW in HVT whereas TUT lasted longer in HIT for all back and chest exercises (t-test, $p = 0.000$), significantly. Overall, a 28 seconds longer TUT with 53 % TW of HVT led to minimal reduction of 1-RM bench press in HIT compared to HVT.

Table 9: Differences of TUT, percentage relation of TW for HIT in % of HVT and also percentage changes in test results for chest and triceps (1-RM bench press)

	1-RM bench press			
subject	**d_{HIT} [%]**	**d_{HVT} [%]**	**$d_{HIT-HVT}$ TUT/TS [sec.]**	**TW HIT in % HVT [kg]**
1	2.17	-4.17	69.14	51.55
2	-4.17	2.13	88.71	57.59
3	-2.00	6.12	30.57	50.81
4	12.20	-4.35	15.29	43.39
5	-8.33	0.00	-20.57	53.40
6	0.00	2.04	-15.00	58.55
mean	-0.02±6.99	0.3±4.05	28.02±44.17	52.55±5.48
d = difference, TS = training session				

3-RM pull-ups showed similar results in HIT with 17 seconds longer TUT per training session and 56 % TW of HVT.

Table 10: Differences of TUT, percentage relation of TW for HIT in % of HVT and also percentage changes in test results for back and biceps muscles (3-RM pull-ups)

	3-RM pull-ups			
subject	d_{HIT} [%]	d_{HVT} [%]	$d_{HIT-HVT}$ TUT/TS [sec.]	TW HIT in % HVT [kg]
1	6.25	5.52	32.29	42.72
2	0.73	5.76	43.43	56.23
3	1.40	3.00	30.86	49.00
4	0.50	-0.65	-0.14	52.62
5	-2.00	2.15	-13.29	54.86
6	1.26	-7.51	8.43	78.51
mean	1.36±2.7	1.38±4.95	16.93±21.95	55.66±12.2
d = difference, TS = training session				

Individual test results identified no homogenous tendency for subjects. Subjects 5 and 6 achieved a performance decrement or preservation with shorter TUT for 1-RM bench press, respectively. Subjects 2 and 3 impaired with distinctly longer TUT whereas subjects 1 and 4 showed better test results with longer TUT.

For 3-RM pull-ups, subjects 4 and 5 displayed a little performance decrement with shorter TUT in HIT. All other subjects increased larger in HIT than HVT with longer TUT. Means of TUT and differences in test results of knee extension and flexion showed performance losses in HIT with longer TUT than in HVT (see table 11 and 12).

In knee extension, average TUT per training session was 10.45 seconds significant longer (t-test, p = 0.011). In both training regimes performance decrements were noticeable. Decrements were higher in HIT (2.42 %) than in HVT (0.57 %) though the difference was not significant (wilcoxon-test, p = 0.480). Only subject 1 improved in both training regimes.

Table 11: Differences of TUT, percentage relation of TW for HIT in % of HVT and also percentage changes in test results of knee extension

	knee extension			
subject	d_{HIT} [%]	d_{HVT} [%]	$d_{HIT-HVT}$ TUT/TS [sec.]	TW HIT in % HVT [kg]
1	7.96	1.87	6.57	48.52
2	-5.02	0.20	37.43	62.50
3	-7.14	-4.19	12.57	49.89
4	6.08	-0.74	20.14	59.35
5	5.69	5.12	-17.71	52.62
6	1.46	-5.69	3.71	63.36
mean	2.42±5.93	-0.57±3.96	10.45±18.33	56.04±6.52
d = difference, TS = training session				

Knee flexion showed an average performance loss of 1.09 % in HIT whereas HVT increased about 3.16 %. This differences between HIT and HVT were not significant (wilcoxon-test, p = 0.248), also average TUT showed no significant differences (t-test, p = 0.098).

Table 12: Differences of TUT, percentage relation of TW for HIT in % of HVT and also percentage changes in test results of knee flexion

	knee flexion			
subject	**d_{HIT} [%]**	**d_{HVT} [%]**	**$d_{HIT-HVT}$ TUT/TS [sec.]**	**TW HIT in % HVT [kg]**
1	0.36	2.58	33.14	45.26
2	-0.65	7.03	58.00	57.86
3	-13.13	7.67	21.43	42.24
4	0.73	-3.14	-8.14	53.17
5	-6.17	4.57	-24.43	53.22
6	12.31	0.26	-1.57	55.60
mean	-1.09±8,44	3.16±4.14	13.07±30.21	51.22±6.12
d = difference, TS = training session				

Noticeably, subject 5 decreased in knee extension and flexion in HIT with evidently shorter TUT than in HVT.

Subject 5 and 6 increased in knee extension with longer TUT in HIT while subject 2, 3 and 4 impaired with longer TUT and extremely swaying TW.

For knee flexion, subjects 4 and 6 showed small to average increases with minimal shorter TUT. Longer TUT and swaying TW led to performance losses or preservation in subjects 1, 2 and 3, respectively.

Regarding all test results, HIT showed a decline of 0.54 % whereas HVT increased with 1.07 %. The difference between performance changes in HIT and HVT was not significant (t-test, p = 0.174). Average TUT was in HIT with 17.12 seconds significant longer (t-test, p = 0.000). Figure 3 displays the important developments.

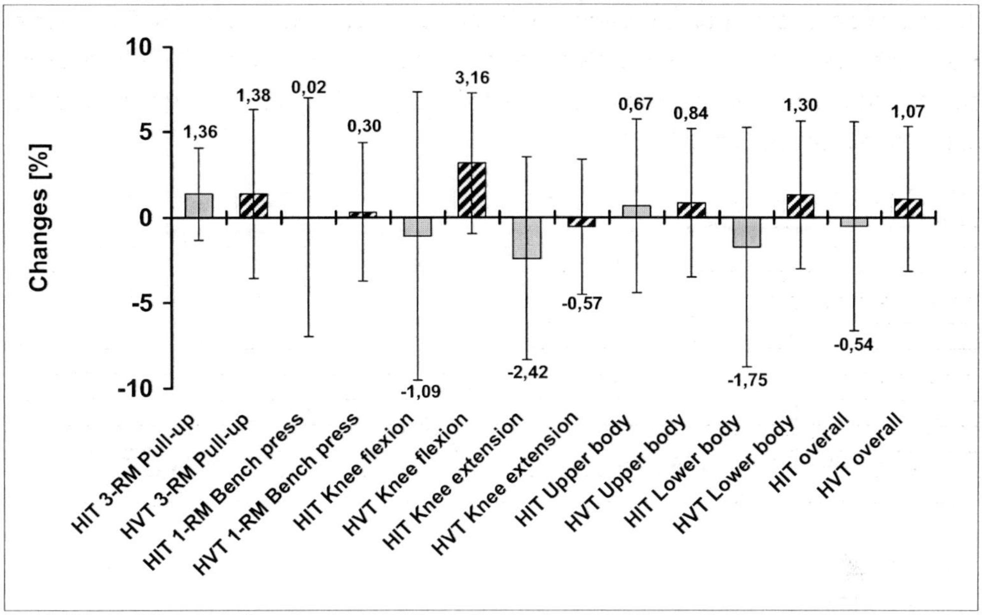

Figure 3: Percentages of changes in test results for HIT (□) and HVT (■)

Discussion

Duration of training sessions

Time saving of low volume HIT was significant but unexpected small (see table 4). There are two possible explanations for this finding. On the one hand, more warm-up sets than training sets were performed. On the other hand, the high-intensity training stress requires longer rest intervals between exercises. Therefore, duration of training sessions in HIT will be influenced by individual recreation capacity between exercises and the number of warm-up sets. For further investigations the author calls the extensive warm-up used in this study into question.

Changes in lean body mass

Comparison of post-tests for both training regimes showed higher lean body mass (see figure 3) for all subjects after HIT than HVT. Lesser LBM after HVT could be related to double training volume. Proponents of low-volume training suggest that high training volume could led to a systemic catabolic condition with delayed muscle hypertrophy and occurred muscle atrophy (Johnston, 2000, p. 126; Kelso, 2000, p. 78; Kieser, 2000, p. 41; Mentzer, 1995, p. 50; Pipes, 1988, p. 109). In addition to local muscular effects, training stimuli also have a systemic/global effect on the whole body (see Johnston, 2000, p. 126). Carpinelli and Otto (1998, p. 84) claim that high training volume causes no adaptations in terms of muscle hypertrophy and strength gains. However, only the number of tolerable training sets will be increased.

Time under tension and total work

Time under tension and total work may play an important role in evaluating changes in test results. Tables 9 to 13 show many aggravations of test outcomes. These developments can be interpreted as misdirected training. Key reasons could be too high or low training stimuli with inadequate time under tension or total work, respectively. There is obviously an optimal range of these two parameters. Because all subjects show half total work in HIT, time under tension could be more prominent than total work. In this context, O'Bryant, Byrd and Stone (1988, p. 29) considered the manipulation of intensity as a prominent factor in their study:

> "These observations support the concept that intensity and its proper manipulation are more important factors (compared to volume) in increasing the 1-RM squat."

Results of this study cast doubt on total work, understood as high number of sets, as primarily stimulus for strength gains and muscle hypertrophy, respectively. However, time under tension may represent another important factor to regulate training volume in strength training.

The time under tension provides a detailed report of physiological stimuli on the trained muscle. Slower repetition speed and use of high-intensity training techniques in HIT indicate longer time under tension - independent of number of sets! Therefore, performance losses in HIT could be the result of a training stimulus set too high. Overall, the effectiveness of low training volume in terms of total work seems to be evident.

In this study, sequence effects (see Zatsiorsky, 1996, p. 31) of training regimes were not controlled but may have influenced the results. Further studies should match sequences.

Individual case analysis subject 1

Individual case analysis purposes the opportunity to identify individual results similar to different recreation needs and adaptations to strength training programs, respectively (see methods). Subject 1 serves as example for analysis of the 1-RM bench press and the training exercises.

As shown in table 9, subject 1 improved his 1-RM bench press about 2.17 % in HIT whereas his performance decreased around 4 % in HVT. Contrary to group tendencies, half total work of HVT with evidently higher time under tension in HIT led to increases in 1-RM bench press after HIT. Individual time under tension for subject 1 (69.14 seconds) showed a 28.02 seconds longer time as groups means. Therefore time under tension may have meaningful importance in increasing muscular strength and inducing muscle hypertrophy, respectively.

Performance losses in HVT could be explained through high training volume that led to overtraining as a result of insufficient adaptation capacities. Another possibility is the lesser mean time under tension in HVT group, corresponding with lesser physiological muscle strain.

Table 13: Comparison of lean body mass (LBM) and fat mass (FM) in HIT and HVT for subject 1

	LBM		FM	
	HIT	HVT	HIT	HVT
pre-test [kg]	58.90	62.17	22.90	19.63
post-test [kg]	62.02	60.34	19.58	23.46
$d_{pre\text{-}post}$ [kg]	3.12	-1.83	-3.32	3.83
$d_{pre\text{-}post}$ [%]	5.30	2.94	14.50	19.51
d = difference, post = post-test, pre = pre-test				

Anthropometric changes in table 13 support the analysis of training parameters. The increase of lean body mass in HIT reflects an optimal training stimulus whereas the loss of lean body mass in HVT indicates deficient strength training. It can be summarized that HIT represents an effective strength training regime to increase 1-RM bench press for subject 1. On the other side HVT needs modifications of total work and time under tension to ensure positive training adaptations. Contrary to group comparisons with no differences between 1-RM bench press for both training regimes, individual case analysis identifies HIT as more effective for subject 1.

Conclusion and practical application

Currently on consideration of the little sample size (n = 6), tendentious recommendations for designing resistance training programs will be presented with regard to training volume. At this HIT will be focused because only a few studies considered this training regime.

Basic modifications of resistance training variables in Low-volume training or HIT, respectively, are number of exercises, high-intensity training techniques and training frequency. Changes in training variables are generally required if the preceding program failed to show the desired performance gains. Table 14 displays a low-volume training program based on the results of this study. Due to supposedly too high training stimuli, training volume is clearly reduced. Pilot studies already showed positive results with anticipated time and performance gains.

Table 14: Modification of LVT including exercises, number of sets and repetitions as well as high-intensity training techniques and time under tension

	exercises	sets x repetitions + HITT	TUT [sec.]
workout 1: HIT	leg extension	1 x 10 - 12 + B	60 - 90
	leg press	1 x 10 - 12 + A	90 - 120
	lying leg curl	1 x 10 - 12 + Iso	60 - 90
	bend over calf raise	1 x 10 - 12 + B	60 - 90
	pull-ups	1 x 8 - 10 + Iso	40 - 60
	machine flies	1 x 8 - 10 + Iso	40 - 60
	dumbell side raise	1 x 8 - 10 + P	40 - 60
	butterly reverse	1 x 8 - 10 + Iso	40 - 60
	cable pushdowns	1 x 8 - 10 + P	40 - 60
	dumbell concentration curl	1 x 8 - 10 + Iso	40 - 60
	hyperextension	1 x 10 - 12 + Iso/B/Iso	60 - 90
	pelvis lift	1 x max.	60 - 90
	crunches	1 x max.	60 - 90
	side bridge	1 x max.	60 - 90
workout 2: SST	leg extension	1 x 10 - 12	60 - 90
	squat	1 x 10 - 12	90 - 120
	seated leg curl	1 x 10 - 12	60 - 90
	stiffed-leg deadlift	1 x 8 - 10	60 - 90
	standing calf raise	1 x 10 - 12	60 - 90
	bent over barbell row	1 x 8 - 10	40 - 60
	bench press	1 x 8 - 10	40 - 60
	dumbell shoulder press	1 x 8 - 10	40 - 60
	dumbell bent over side raise	1 x 8 - 10	40 - 60
	french press	1 x 8 - 10	40 - 60
	barbell curl	1 x 8 - 10	40 - 60
	pelvis lift	1 x max.	60 - 90
	crunches	1 x max.	60 - 90
	side bridge	1 x max.	60 - 90

A = assisted positive repetition, B = breakdown set, Iso = isometric contraction, max. = maximum repetitions, P = partial repetitions, HITT = high-intensity training technique, TuT = time under tension, SST = single-set training

The number of exercises is reduced to one exercise per muscle group. So a whole body workout instead of a split program is possible. In order to avoid overtraining, intensity of exertion (see also Brzycki, 1995, p. 35; Philipp, 1999b, p. 31) varies from one training session to another.

Training 1 represents a HIT and applies various high-intensity training techniques. Only one high-intensity training techniques per exercise is used. Training 2 displays a single-set training, per definition without any high-intensity training techniques. For both trainings programs it is crucial to achieve the necessary time under tension for each muscle group. Depending on training status 2 to 3 training sessions per week are sufficient, especially under consideration of other training contents.

Furthermore not all exercises are suitable for HIT, particularly coordinative demanding multi-joint free weight exercises. Maintaining perfect form becomes difficult with progressing muscular fatigue and exertion so that injury risk may increase. Additional, small synergistic muscle groups exhaust first and the primary target muscle group achieves not the desired training effect.

Consequentially, training 1 (HIT) uses training machines to assure a safe and direct overload of the target muscles. Because of a lower intensity of exertion, Training 2 (SST) includes free weight exercises.

A composite list of exercise selection is useful to design sport-specific training programs. Hence, exercises can be chosen under specific and functional criterions.

Regarding changes in body composition and strength in experienced fitness athletes this study shows no differences between a high-volume training program and a low-volume training program. These observations - under consideration of the small sample size - call common training recommendations and widespread practices into question.

Training data and test results do not suggest that low volume high-intensity training represents an insufficient training stimulus in highly trained athletes. In fact, the opposite seems to be true: the immense effectiveness of HIT requires distinctive care in designing high-intensity training programs. In order to avoid symptoms of overtraining, infrequent training (longer recreation phases) and brief training sessions (inverse relationship between intensity and duration) are recommended.

It can be summarized that Low-volume training (SST and HIT) represents an efficient training regime that still needs further research. An evaluation of long term training adaptations, usage of periodization and utilization in rehabilitation and high performance training should be focussed on.

References

Baechle, T. R., Earle, R., & Wathen, D. (2000). Resistance training. In T. R. Baechle & R. Earle (Eds.), *Essentials of strength training and conditioning* (pp. 395-425). Champaign, IL: Human Kinetics.

Boeckh-Behrens, W.-U., & Buskies, W. (2000). *Fitness-Krafttraining [Fitness strength training]* (1st ed.). Reinbek bei Hamburg: Rowohlt.

Brzycki, M. (1995). *A practical approach to strength training* (3rd ed.). Lincolnwood: Masters Press.

Brzycki, M. (1998). *The REPS prescription will help your clients remember basics of strength training movements for greater effectiveness and safety.* Retrieved July, 2001, from http://www.fitnessmanagement.com/info/fr/articles.html

Carpinelli, R. N., & Otto, R. M. (1998). Strength training. Single versus multiple sets. *Sports Medicine, 26*(2), 73-84.

Fleck, S. J., & Kraemer, W. J. (2004). *Designing resistance training programs* (3rd ed.). Champaign, IL: Human Kinetics.

Gießing, J. (2000). Das Heavy-Duty-Konzept. Zunehmende Akzeptanz und Popularität des Einsatz-Trainings auch beim Bodybuilding [The Heavy-Duty-Concept. Increasing acceptance and popularity of single-set training in bodybuilding]. *Leistungssport, 30*(4), 19-23.

Gießing, J. (2003). Training for muscular hypertrophy: A comparison of high and low-volume approaches. *International Journal of Physical Education, 15*(1), 27-32.

Gießing, J., Preuss, P., Greiwing, A., Goebel, S., Müller, A., Schischek, A. & Stephan, A. (2005). Fundamental definitions of decisive training parameters of single-set training and multiple-set training for muscular hypertrophy. In J. Gießing, M. Fröhlich & P. Preuss (Eds.), *Current results in strength training research. An empirical and theoretical approach* (pp. 9-23). Göttingen: Cuvillier.

Harrison, C. (2000). In search of the perfect program. In M. Brzycki (Ed.), *Maximize your training: insights from leading strength and fitness professionals* (pp. 97-113). Lincolnwood, IL: Masters Press.

Hass, C. J., Garzarella, L., de Hoyos, D., & Pollock, M. L. (2000). Single versus multiple sets in long-term recreational weightlifters. *Medicine & Science in Sports & Exercise, 32*(1), 235-242.

Heiduk, R., Preuss, P., & Steinhöfer, D. (2002). Die optimale Satzzahl im Krafttraining: Einsatz- versus Mehrsatz-Training [The optimal number of sets: single-set versus multiple-set training]. *Leistungssport, 32*(4), 4-13.

Johnston, B. D. (2000). High intensity versus high volume. In M. Brzycki (Ed.), *Maximize your training: insights from leading strength and fitness professionals* (pp. 125-143). Lincolnwood, IL: Masters Press.

Kelso, T. (2000). The basics of muscle contraction: implications for strength training. In M. Brzycki (Ed.), *Maximize your training: insights from leading strength and fitness professionals* (pp. 35-80). Lincolnwood, IL: Master Press.

Kemmler, W., Lauber, D., Engelke, K., & Weineck, J. (2004). Effects of single- vs. multiple-set resistance training on maximum strength and body composition in trained postmenopausal women. *Journal of Strength and Conditioning Research, 18*(4), 689-694.

Kieser, W. (1998). Wieviele Sätze beim Krafttraining? Theorie und Praxis [How much sets in strength training? Theory and practice]. *Leistungssport, 28*(3), 50-51.

Kieser, W. (2000). *Ein starker Rücken kennt keinen Schmerz. Gesundheitsorientiertes Krafttraining nach der Kieser-Methode [A strong back knows no pain. Health orientated strength training according to the Kieser-Method].* München: Heyne.

Mentzer, M. (1995). *Heavy duty.* Heilbronn: Sport Verlag.

O'Bryant, H. S., Byrd, R. J., & Stone, M. H. (1988). Cycle ergometer performance and maximum leg and hip strength adaptations to two different methods of weight training. *Journal of Applied Sport Psychology* 2(2), 27-30.

Paulsen, G., Myklestad, D., & Raastad, T. (2003). The influence of volume of exercise on early adaptations to strength training. *Journal of Strength and Conditioning Research, 17*(1), 115-120.

Peterson, M. D., Rhea, M. R., & Alvar, B. A. (2004). Maximizing strength development in athletes: a meta-analysis to determine the dose-response relationship. *Journal of Strength and Conditioning Research, 18*(2), 377-382.

Philipp, M. (1999a). Ein Satz genügt! - Erfahrungen mit Mehrsatz- und Einsatz-Methoden im Krafttraining. Eine Fallstudie als Diskussionsbeitrag zur Anregung von Werner Kieser [One set is enough! - Experiences with multilpe-set and single-set training in strength training. A case study to adress the controversy with Werner Kieser]. *Leistungssport, 29*(1), 26-28.

Philipp, M. (1999b). Einsatz-Training versus Mehrsatz-Training. Zur Kontroverse um die Satzzahl beim Krafttraining unter Berücksichtigung empirischer Evidenzen [Single-set versus multiple-set training. To adress the controversy under consideration of empirical data]. *Leistungssport, 29*(4), 27-34.

Pipes, T. V. (1988). A.C.T. - The steroid alternative. *Scholastic Coach, 1*, 106-113.

Remmert, H., Schischek, A., Zamhöfer, T., & Ferrauti, A. (2005). Zum Einfluss der Regenerationsdauer auf die Kraft- und Muskelmassenzunahme im Rahmen eines Einsatz-Hochintensitätstrainings (High-intensity training) [Influence of regeneration period on strength and lean body mass increases in single-set high-intensity training]. *Leistungssport, 35*(2), 15-19.

Rhea, M. R., Alvar, B. A., Ball, S. D., & Burkett, L. N. (2002). Three sets of weight training superior to 1 set with equal intensity for eliciting strength. *Journal of Strength and Conditioning Research, 16*(4), 525-529.

Rhea, M. R., Alvar, B. A., Burkett, L. N., & Ball, S. D. (2003). A meta-analysis to determine the dose response for strength development. *Medicine & Science in Sports & Exercise, 35*(3), 456-464.

Schlicht, W. (1988). *Einzelfallanalysen im Hochleistungssport: zum Verlauf und zur Wirkung selbstbezogener Aufmerksamkeit im 400-Meter-Hürdenlauf [Single case analysis in high performance sport: course and effect of self-orientated attentiveness in 400-m-hurdles]*: Schorndorf: Hofmann.

Schlumberger, A., & Schmidtbleicher, D. (1999). Einsatz-Training als trainingsmethodische Alternative - Möglichkeiten und Grenzen [Single-set training as methodical alternative - potentials and limits]. *Leistungssport, 29*(3), 9-11.

Schlumberger, A., Stec, J., & Schmidtbleicher, D. (2001). Single- vs. multiple-set strength training in women. *Journal of Strength and Conditioning Research, 15*(3), 284-289.

Szubski, C. (1999). Der Einsatz-Training versus Mehrsatz-Training-Dogmatismus - Ein Beispiel für Glaubenslehren in der Trainingswissenschaft? [The single-set versus multiple-set dogmatism - an example for dogma in sport science?]. *Leistungssport, 29*(4), 35.

Tan, B. (1999). Manipulating resistance training program variables to optimize maximum strength in men: a review. *Journal of Strength and Conditioning Research, 13*(3), 289-304.

Weingarten, S. (2000). Bodybuilding HIT. In M. Brzycki (Ed.), *Maximize your training: insights from leading strength and fitness professionals* (pp. 319-334). Lincolnwood, IL: Masters Press.

Westcott, W. L., Winett, R. A., Anderson, E. S., Wojcik, J. R., Loud, R. L., Cleggett, E., et al. (2001). Effects of regular and slow speed resistance training on muscle strength. *Journal of Sports Medicine and Physical Fitness, 41*(2), 154-158.

Winett, R. A. (2004). Meta-analyses do not support performance of multiple sets or high volume resistance training. *Journal of Exercise Physiology online, 7*(5), 10-20.

Wolfe, B. L., LeMura, L. M., & Cole, P. J. (2004). Quantitative analysis of single- vs. multiple-set programs in resistance training. *Journal of Strength and Conditioning Research, 18*(1), 35-47.

Wolfe, B. L., Valerio, T. A., Strohecker, K., & Szmedra, L. (2001). Effect of single versus multiple-set resistance training on muscular strength. *Medicine & Sciene in Sports & Exercise, 33*(5), S76.

Yates, D., & Wolff, B. (1995). *Blut und Schweiss. Die ultimative Methode zum Aufbau maximaler Muskelmasse [Blood and guts. The ultimate approach to building maximum muscle mass]*. Heilbronn: Sport-Verlag, Ingenohl.

Zatsiorsky, V. M. (1996). *Krafttraining - Wissenschaft und Praxis [Science and practice of strength training]*. Aachen: Meyer & Meyer.

ANDREAS GREIWING & JÜRGEN FREIWALD

Effects of three resistance training methods on maximal strength, strength endurance and muscle thickness of the m. quadriceps femoris

(Project "Strength Training Methods" - BISP Reference VF0407/05/42/2003-2004)

Keywords: single-set training, multiple-set training, high-intensity training, muscular hypertrophy, time series design

Introduction

It is well known that resistance training is the most effective method available for improving muscle strength and lean body mass (Atha, 1981; Fleck & Kraemer, 2004; Hollmann, Hettinger, & Strüder, 2000; Kraemer & Häkkinen, 2002). By variation of the acute program variables an almost indefinite number of strength training programs can be created (Fleck & Kraemer, 2004, p. 158). The importance of one of the acute program variables, the training volume (total number of repetitions performed during a training session multiplied by the resistance used) for the efficiency of a resistance training program, is still unclear. Low volume and high volume approaches are used in recreational fitness settings, but also in professional sports to increase strength, power and muscle mass (ACSM, 1998; Ebben & Blackard, 2001; Feigenbaum & Pollock, 1997). The single-set training system is an example for the low volume approach, the multiple-set system is a typical high volume approach.

Different definitions of the termini "single-set system" and "multiple-set system" exist. Fleck and Kraemer (2004, pp. 188-189) define the single-set system as "...the performance of each exercise for one set" and the multiple-set system as "virtually any training system that consists of more than one set of an exercise...". In contrast Schlumberger und Schmidtbleicher (1999, p. 9) define single-set training as the execution of only one set per muscle group for a specific exercise. Schlumberger und Schmidtbleicher (1999) do not give an exact definition for multiple-set training, but state that most multiple-set systems incorporate between 3 - 6 sets per exercise with 2 - 3 minutes rest intervals between the sets.

A special low volume approach is the high-intensity training (HIT). HIT is characterized by 1 set per exercise followed by exhaustion techniques to achieve maximum fatigue (Gießing, 2005; Heiduk, Preuss, & Steinhöfer, 2002). Popular examples for exhaustion techniques are forced repetitions in which a partner helps to accomplish one or two extra repetitions after positive muscular fatigue and drop sets in which (after reaching positive fatigue) the weight is immediately reduced by 20 - 25 % and as many additional repetitions as possible are performed (Weingarten, 2000).

Ahtiainen, Pakarinen, Kraemer and Hakkinen (2003) compared the effects of a multiple-set maximum repetition strength training with a multiple-set forced repetitions strength training on hormonal and neuromuscular parameters. Both strength training protocols led to significant ($p < 0.05 - 0.001$) acute increases in serum testosterone, free testosterone, cortisol and growth hormone (GH) concentrations and to significant reductions in maximal isometric force. The multiple-set forced repetitions group showed significantly larger acute cortisol ($p < 0.05$) and GH ($p < 0.01$) concentrations and a larger decrease of maximal isometric force ($p < 0.001$). There are numerous studies comparing the efficiency of multiple-set and single-set resistance training programs to improve muscular strength (Berger, 1962; Hass, Garzarella, de Hoyos, & Pollock, 2000; Jacobson, 1986; Kramer et al., 1997; Marx et al., 2001; Paulsen, Myklestad, & Raastad, 2003; Rhea, Alvar, Ball, & Burkett, 2002; Sanborn et al., 2000; Schlumberger, Stec, & Schmidtbleicher, 2001; Starkey et al., 1996; Stowers, 1983). Though most of the studies cited support the superiority of multiple-set-programs for optimal strength improvements (Berger, 1962; Kraemer, 1997; Marx et al., 2001; Paulsen et al., 2003; Rhea et al., 2002; Sanborn et al., 2000; Schlumberger et al., 2001) a number of studies claim that single-set programs are equally efficient (Hass et al., 2000; Jacobson, 1986; Starkey et al., 1996). In a recently published meta-analysis Wolfe, LeMura, and Cole (2004) compared 16 studies on single-set vs. multiple-set resistance training programs. In a final conclusion the authors recommended ...

> "the use of multiple-set programs for trained individuals and single-set programs for untrained individuals during the initial short training period." (Wolfe et al., 2004, p. 46)

In contrast to the number of studies comparing the efficiency of multiple-set and single-set training programs for the improvement of maximum strength, only few studies evaluate the effects of these training methods on strength endurance and muscular hypertrophy (Hass et al., 2000; Starkey et al., 1996).

Therefore the purpose of our study was to investigate the efficiency of multiple-set, single-set and HIT training programs not only for the improvement of maximum strength, but also for the development of strength endurance and muscular hypertrophy. If single-set and/or HIT resistance training programs would be as effective, or even more effective, as multiple-set resistance training programs, this finding would support these training methods as time efficient alternatives to the traditional time consuming multiple-set program.

Methods

Subjects

Eleven male and eleven female subjects participated in this study (age: 26.86 $\pm$ 5.45; weight: 70.05 $\pm$ 10.04 kg; height: 176.82 $\pm$ 8.70 cm. The subjects had a background of at least 6 month of weight training experience and no injuries or chronic diseases of the lower extremities. 17 subjects were matched for initial maximal isometric strength and randomly assigned to 1 of 3 training groups, 4 subjects were assigned to a control group and 1 subject served as a "control person" (The subject was tested in weekly intervals to detect possible observer effects caused by the test protocol). There were no significant isometric strength differences between the 4 groups ($p < 0.05$; Kruskal-Wallis Test).

Study design

A time series design was used. Prior to the training period a familiarization period of 1 week was implemented. Also, a final test (Post-Test) was conducted after a detraining period of 1 week (see figure 1).

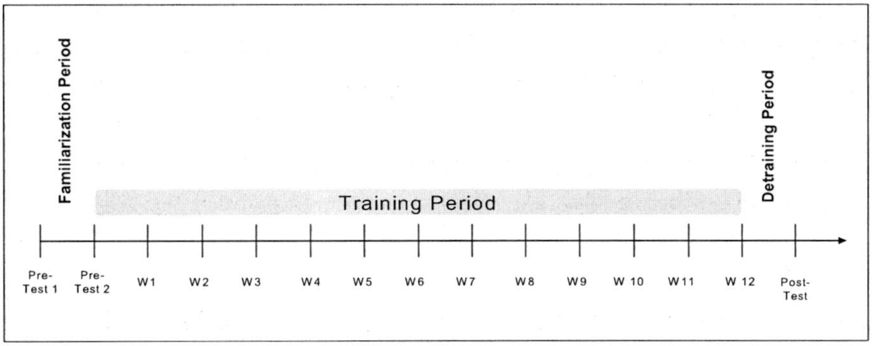

Figure 1: Experimental design of the study. The tests after each training week are labeled W1 (test after training week 1) to W12 (test after training week 12)

Testing

M. quadriceps femoris muscle thickness, isometric strength, and muscular endurance of both legs were measured in weekly intervals after the familiarization period (Pre-Test 2 - Post-Test). An isometric strength test was conducted prior to the familiarization period to determine baseline isometric strength (Pre-Test 1). The tests were carried out in the following order:

1) Ultrasound muscle thickness measurement,
2) Isometric strength test,
3) Body weight and percentage body fat measurements,
4) Strength endurance test.

Ultrasound Muscle Thickness Measurement

The muscle thickness of the m. quadriceps femoris for both legs was measured using a Fukuda Denshi UF-4500 scanner (Fukuda Denshi; Tokyo, Japan) equipped with a 5-MHz linear transducer (FUT-L104). The subjects were placed in a supine position with a cushion under the popliteal fossa of the leg to be scanned. This allowed for a 10° bend of the knee and ensured that the thigh was relaxed (Bemben, 2002, p. 105). Ultrasound scans were conducted at 30 %, 50 % and 70 % the distance from the proximal border of the patella to the spina iliaca superior anterior on the anterior surface of the thigh. The locations were labeled D_{30}, D_{50} and D_{70}. The arithmetic middle of these 3 values was also calculated and labeled as D_{kom}. To ensure precise relocation of the measurement sites permanent skin blemishes and the scanning locations were traced onto a transparent sheet (Dons, Bollerup, Bonde-Petersen, & Hancke, 1979). A liberal amount of ultrasound gel was used to minimize compression of the thigh tissue. As soon as a clear picture, which allowed identification of the femur and the fasziae, was visible on the monitor, the ultrasound device's "freeze option" was activated and the picture was printed by means of a Sony UP 890 CE (Sony; Tokyo, Japan) video printer. The muscle layer (distance between the fat-muscle interface and muscle-bone interface) was measured to the nearest 0.01 mm with a digital caliper (Pollock, Garzarella, & Graves, 1995, p. 192). The reliability and validity of ultrasound scans as a means of muscle hypertrophy assessment is documented (Abe, Kawakami, Suzuki, Gunji, & Fukunaga, 1997; Bemben, 2002).

Isometric Strength

A chair dynamometer was used to determine maximal unilateral isometric strength of both legs. During testing the subject was secured by 1 Velcro strap around the hip and 2 Velcro straps around the thigh, the knee was flexed at 90° (see Figure 2). A non-elastic strap was placed around the leg just above the malleoli. The strap was attached to a load cell (Digimax - Mechatronic; Hamm, Germany) which was connected to a personal computer. On verbal command the subjects were encouraged to gradually increase force against the strap and reach their maximum 2 - 3 seconds after the start of the test. Two trials per leg were conducted, the measurement time for each test was 5 seconds, the rest period between the trials was approximately 30 seconds. The highest recorded value (Newton) was defined as the maximal isometric force.

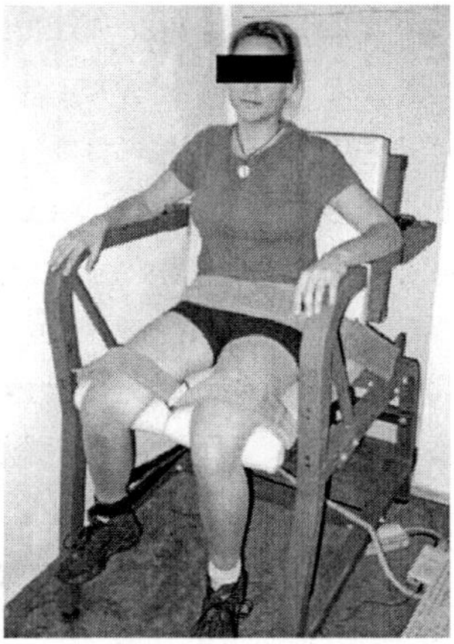

Figure 2: Isometric strength test

Strength Endurance

The strength endurance test was conducted on a leg extension machine (Schnell; Peutenhausen, Germany). A strong correlation between the isometric tests on the chair dynamometer and the 1-repetition-maximum on the leg extension machine ($p < 0.001$; $\tau = 0{,}969$ Kendall´s Tau Correlation) allowed strength endurance testing based on the isometric strength test. The resistance chosen for strength endurance testing was approximately 34 % of the maximum dynamic strength. Repetition number was defined as strength endurance. The subjects were instructed to complete the concentric and eccentric phase of the leg extension exercise in 1 second each.

Body weight and percentage body fat

Body weight and percentage body fat were determined with a Tanita TBF-300 (Tanita; Sindelfingen, Germany) body fat analyzer. This device utilizes leg-to-leg bioelectrical impedance analysis (BIA) to assess body composition.

Training

The strength training consisted of 6 exercises:

- leg extension (unilateral),
- leg curl (unilateral),
- bench press,
- lateral pull-down,
- abdominal crunch,
- back extension.

All treatment groups trained 3 times per week. During the 1 week familiarization period the subjects performed 3 sets with 12 - 15 repetitions not to exhaustion, but until their perceived exertion reached intensity level 5 (middle to heavy) according to the rating of the perceived exertion scale by Boeckh-Behrens and Buskies (2001, p. 75) (A 7 point perceived exertion scale ranging from level 1 (very easy) to level 7 (very hard)).

Throughout the training period all sets were carried out until no further repetition could be accomplished. The movement speed for all exercises was approximately 1 second for the concentric phase and 1 second for the eccentric phase. During the first 6 weeks of the training period 12 - 15 repetitions were performed for each set. During the second 6 weeks of the training period the load was increased so that only 6 - 8 repetitions were possible for each set.

Multiple-Set Protocol (N = 3; male: 2; female: 1)

The multiple-set group performed 3 sets per exercise for all 6 exercises. Three sets per leg were conducted for the leg extension and the leg curl. The sets for the right and left leg were alternated. The rest periods between the sets lasted approximately 2 minutes.

Single-Set Protocol (N = 3; male: 2; female: 1)

The single-set group performed 1 set for all 6 exercises. For the leg extension and leg curl exercise 1 set was conducted for each leg. There were no additional rest periods between the exercises.

HIT Protocol (N = 5; male: 2, female: 3)

The subjects of the HIT training group performed 1 set of 12 - 15, respectively 6 - 8 repetitions until exhaustion. Immediately after the last repetition the subject reduced the weight by approximately 20 % and performed as many additional repetitions as possible.

Control Group (N = 4; male: 1; female: 3)

The subjects of the control group did not participate in any form of resistance training and were tested and re-tested within approximately 3 month (mean: 98.25 ± 7.27 days).

Control subject (male)

The subject was tested in weekly intervals to evaluate the influence of the testing sessions (observer effect). He did not participate in any form of resistance training.

Statistical analyses

Because both female and male subjects participated in this study relative (percentage) values were evaluated. The tests by Cox and Stuart (Sachs, 2002, pp. 487-488) and Wallis and Moore (Bortz & Lienert, 2003, pp. 328-332) were used to detect significant trends in the time series. Significant Pre-Test maximal isometric strength differences between the groups were analyzed by means of the Kruskal and Wallis test. In a separate test Kendall's Tau was calculated to identify a possible correlation between maximal isometric strength determined on the chair dynamometer and 1-repetition-maximum on the leg extension machine.
Additionally maximum percentage gains of the 3 parameters muscle thickness, isometric strength, and muscular endurance were analyzed with non-parametric tests (Kruskall and Wallis test, Wilcoxon test, cf. Bortz & Lienert 2003). The parameters muscle thickness, isometric strength and strength en-

durance were recorded and analyzed separately for each leg. Statistical significance was accepted at $p < 0.05$.

Results

16 subjects completed the study. 6 subjects (treatment groups) were excluded because of injuries (1 subject - injury not related to the study) and not attending a minimum of 85 % of the training sessions (5 subjects). The percent values presented in the following figures represent the percentage mean values of the groups.

Muscle Thickness

Figure 3 illustrates the combined D_{Kom} values in percent. The Cox and Stuart test indicates significant positive trends for the multiple-set and the single-set group, but not for the HIT group ($p < 0.05$). The Wallis and Moore test indicates no significant trend for any of the analyzed time series.

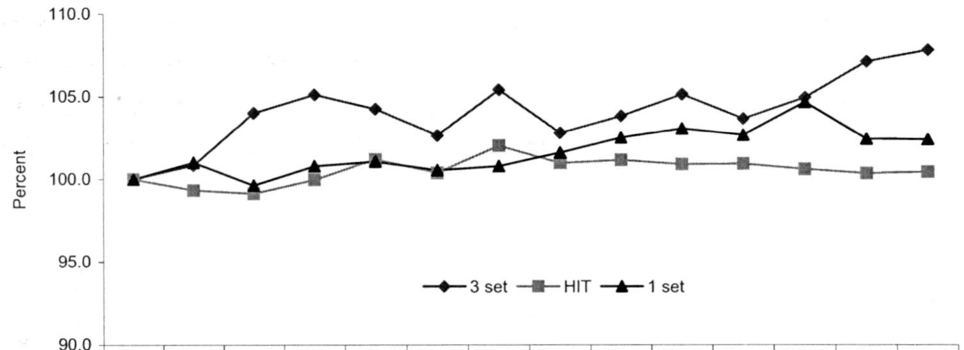

	Pre-Test 2	Week 1	Week 2	Week 3	Week 4	Week 5	Week 6	Week 7	Week 8	Week 9	Week 10	Week 11	Week 12	Post Test
3 set	100.00	100.83	104.01	105.11	104.25	102.63	105.40	102.79	103.82	105.12	103.64	104.93	107.12	107.82
HIT	100.00	99.327	99.128	99.961	101.19	100.38	102.01	100.96	101.14	100.89	100.91	100.59	100.34	100.44
1 set	100.00	101.00	99.626	100.77	101.05	100.53	100.77	101.59	102.50	103.04	102.66	104.65	102.42	102.39

Figure 3: Muscle thickness development (in percent)

Isometric Strength

Figure 4 shows the isometric strength development of the 3 treatment groups. The Cox and Stuart test indicates a significant positive trend only for the multiple-set group ($p < 0.05$). The Wallis and Moore test indicates trends for the multiple and the single-set group ($p < 0.05$).

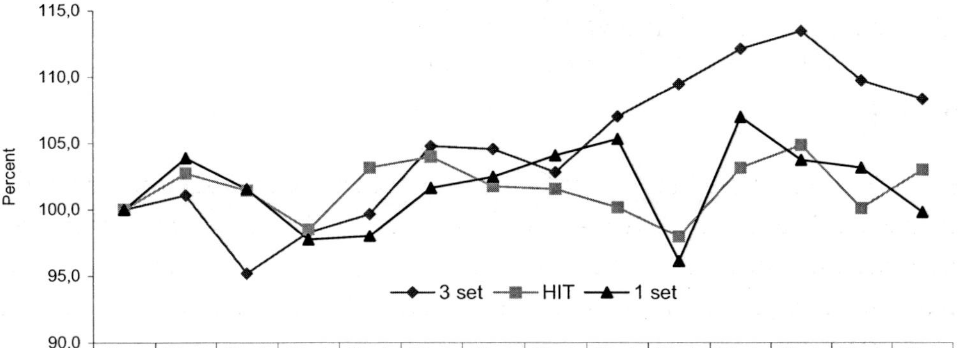

	Pre-Test 2	Week 1	Week 2	Week 3	Week 4	Week 5	Week 6	Week 7	Week 8	Week 9	Week 10	Week 11	Week 12	Post Test
3 set	100,00	101,08	95,21	98,28	99,67	104,78	104,54	102,81	106,99	109,46	112,12	113,46	109,73	108,32
HIT	100,00	102,73	101,44	98,50	103,16	103,98	101,75	101,54	100,17	97,96	103,15	104,86	100,11	103,00
1 set	100,00	103,90	101,52	97,72	97,99	101,61	102,47	104,06	105,32	96,12	106,95	103,75	103,17	99,81

Figure 4: Isometric strength development (in percent)

Strength Endurances

Figure 5 demonstrates the strength endurance development of the 3 training groups. Both trend tests indicate significant positive trends for all 3 treatment groups with the exception of the Wallis and Moore test for the strength endurance development of the single-set group. The subjects completed between 10 to 55 repetitions (mean value of all trials and all treatment groups: 29.55 ± 4.37).

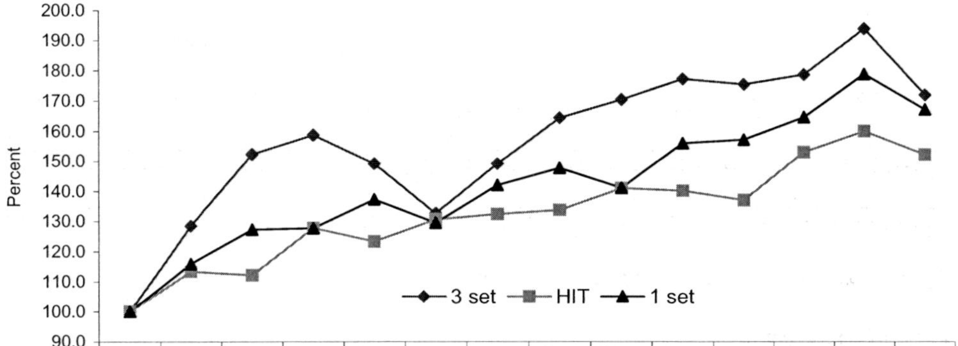

	Pre-Test 2	Week 1	Week 2	Week 3	Week 4	Week 5	Week 6	Week 7	Week 8	Week 9	Week 10	Week 11	Week 12	Post Test
3 set	100.00	128.48	152.33	158.66	149.16	132.70	149.16	164.40	170.41	177.25	175.42	178.63	193.76	171.97
HIT	100.00	113.35	112.20	127.80	123.30	130.66	132.39	133.73	141.04	140.16	137.05	152.96	159.97	152.14
1 set	100.00	115.91	127.35	127.77	137.24	129.54	141.98	147.71	141.12	155.95	157.12	164.56	178.84	167.12

Figure 5: Strength endurance development (in percent)

Maximal changes of the three main parameters muscle thickness, isometric strength and strength endurance

The following table summarizes the maximal changes for the 3 main parameter muscle thickness, isometric strength and strength endurance between the Pre-Test 2 values and the maximal changes (Wilcoxon test). Statistical comparisons (Kruskal and Wallis tests) between the treatment groups showed no significant differences.

*Table 1: Maximal muscle thickness, isometric strength and strength endurance changes (in percent) (*sig. different from Pre-Test 2 value ($p < 0.05$); **sig. different from Pre-Test 2 value ($p < 0.01$)*

group	muscle thickness (D_{Kom})	isometric strength	strength endurance
3 set	+7.82 ± 6.36*	+13.46 ± 6.42*	+93.76 ± 101.98*
HIT	+2.01 ± 3.69	+4.86 ±10.88	+59.98 ± 38.31**
1 set	+4.65 ± 3.87	+6.95 ± 10.95*	+78.85 ± 87.95*
control group	-1.57 ± 3.73	-1.23 ± 4.58	+3.55 ± 7.48

Maximal body weight and percentage body fat changes

Because of the low number of subjects only descriptive statistics of the maximal percentage changes for body weight and percentage body fat are presented in table 2.

Table 2: Maximal body weight and percentage body fat changes (in percent) (⁺percentage change in relation to Pre-Test 2 values)

group	body weight	percentage body fat⁺
3 set	+ 1.48 ± 1.33	+ 7.51 ± 3.70
HIT	+ 0.77 ± 1.08	+ 4.20 ± 6.75
1 set	+ 2.03 ± 0.32	+ 12.46 ± 14.30
control group	- 2.20 ± 2.30	- 6.32 ± 7.88

Control person

Trend analysis shows no significant changes for the parameter muscle thickness, isometric strength and strength endurance for the combined values of both legs. However, combined strength endurance increased by 52.08 ± 26.52 percent and individual analysis of the strength endurance changes for each leg indicates a significant positive trend for the left leg (Cox and Stuart; $p < 0.05$).

Discussion

The results oft his study indicate the superiority of the higher volume multiple-set program for increasing muscle thickness, maximal isometric strength, and strength endurance of the m. quadriceps femoris. The multiple-set group improves the most for all 3 parameters, followed by the single-set group and the HIT group.

The maximal muscle thickness gains of the multiple-set group (+7.82 ± 6.36) are almost twice as high as the gains of the single-set group (+4.65 ± 3.87) and more than 3 times the improvement of the HIT group (+2.01 ± 3.69). Even though the Cox and Stuart test shows a significant positive trend for the multiple-set and the single-set group, only the maximal muscle thickness change of the multiple-set group shows a significant improvement from Pre-Test 2 values. Abe, DeHoyos, Pollock and Garzarella (2000) have reported muscle thickness gains of 7 % (m. quadriceps femoris, at 50 % thigh length between the lateral condyle of the femur and greater trochanter, starting at the greater trochanter) in untrained men and women after 12 weeks of single- and multiple-set resistance training. Interestingly, not only the maximal gains, but also the time course of the muscle thickness changes in the study of Abe et al. (2000) are quite similar to the muscle thickness changes in our study (see Abe et al. 2000, p. 178).

Similar to the muscle thickness changes, maximal isometric gains of the multiple-set group (+13.46 ± 6.42) are almost twice as high as the single- set group (+6.95 ± 10.95) and almost 3 times as high as the HIT group (+4.86 ± 10.88). The isometric strength gains of the single-set group in our study is in agreement with the reported isometric strength gains of the single-set group (+6.3 %) reported in the study by Hass et al. (2000). 42 trained male and female subjects trained 3 times per week for 13 weeks. They completed a resistance training circuit once (single-set) or 3 times (multiple-set). The subjects conducted 8 - 12 repetitions to muscular failure.

However, Hass et al. (2000) reported only a 6.8 % isometric strength gain for the multiple-set group in their study, which is far less than the 13.46 % gain of our study. The reason for this divergent result may be the design of the multiple-set program in the study by Hass et al. (2000). In contrast to our study Hass et al. (2000) used a circuit design, not a sequence of 3 sets of 1 exercise, as in our study.

The strength endurance gains were much larger than the isometric strength gains or the muscle thickness gains. Even though the multiple-set group achieved the largest gains, all groups showed significant improvements in the time series analysis and in comparison between maximal gains to Pre-Test 2 values. The magnitude of the strength endurance improvements is lower as in the earlier mentioned study by Hass et al. (2000), but the strength endurance test in that study was conducted with 75 % of the 1-repetition-maximum in contrast to approximately 34 % of the 1-repetition maximum used in our study. The control person, who was tested in weekly intervals, increased his strength endurance significantly (Cox and Stuart) by 70.83 % for his left leg and 33.33 % (not significant) for his right leg. These results raise the question if a traditional multiple-set training is necessary to improve muscular endurance. One testing session per week of one set performed with a relative low percentage of the 1-RM (approximately 34 % of 1-RM) seemed to be sufficient to induce major strength endurance improvements. Because this finding is based on only one person it has to be interpreted with caution.
The presented body weight and percentage body fat alterations (see table 2) have to be interpreted with caution. Nutrition was not controlled so it is not certain whether the reported changes were caused by the different training methods. Additionally, the accuracy of leg-to-leg bioelectrical impedance analysis for the assessment of body fat alterations is still discussed (Herm, 2003) and the absolute body weight and percentage body fat changes for the treatment groups measured in this study were small (maximum mean weight change [single-set group]: +1.27 $\pm$ 0.12 kg; maximum mean body fat change [multiple-set group]: +1.43 $\pm$ 1.16 %). Nevertheless, only the multiple-set group showed a significant positive trend for the parameter body weight and percentage body fat (Cox and Stuart).

Practical Applications

Our study supports the importance of training volume for optimal strength and hypertrophy adaptations. This finding is in accordance with recent meta-analyses on the efficiency of multiple-set and single-set training systems (Rhea, Alvar, Burkett, & Ball, 2003; Wolfe et al., 2004). Even though the multiple-set group improved their strength endurance the most, it is doubtful if the difference between the multiple-set and single-set group would be of any practical importance for the parameter strength endurance. The results of the control person raise the question if optimal strength endurance gains are possible with a vastly reduced training frequency.

Interestingly the HIT group showed the smallest gains of all the treatment groups. Apparently the succession of 2 sets without a sufficient rest period led to higher physiological stress than the other 2 training methods (see Ahtiainen et al., 2003). If HIT systems are to be used, longer recovery periods than the ones required for multiple-set and single-set systems might be necessary. Multiple-set systems should be employed if maximal strength and hypertrophy gains are the training goal and time is not a limiting factor. The time efficiency of single-set programs might be an important factor for subjects who need to combine a resistance training program for example with an endurance program.

Despite the vast amount of information regarding the influence of training volume on maximal strength development, there is still a lack of research on the influence of training volume on muscle hypertrophy. Paulsen et al. (2003) showed in their study that a single-set system was equally effective as a multiple-set system for the training of upper body muscles, but not for the lower body muscles. Future studies should clarify the question whether single-set systems are equally effective as multiple-set systems to stimulate muscle hypertrophy not only for the m. quadriceps femoris, but also for other muscles.

References

Abe, T., DeHoyos, D. V., Pollock, M. L., & Garzarella, L. (2000). Time course for strength and muscle thickness changes following upper and lower body resistance training in men and women. *European Journal of Applied Physiology, 81*(3), 174-180.

Abe, T., Kawakami, Y., Suzuki, Y., Gunji, A., & Fukunaga, T. (1997). Effects of 20 days bed rest on muscle morphology. *Journal of Gravitational Physiology, 4*(1), S10-14.

ACSM. (1998). The recommended quantity and quality of exercise for developing and maintaining cardiorespiratory and muscular fitness, and flexibility in healthy adults. *Medicine & Science in Sports & Exercise, 30*(6), 975-991.

Ahtiainen, J. P., Pakarinen, A., Kraemer, W. J., & Hakkinen, K. (2003). Acute hormonal and neuromuscular responses and recovery to forced vs maximum repetitions multiple resistance exercises. *International Journal of Sports Medicine, 24*(6), 410-418.

Atha, J. (1981). Strengthening muscle. *Exercise and Sport Sciences Reviews, 9*, 1-73.

Bemben, M. G. (2002). Use of diagnostic ultrasound for assessing muscle size. *Journal of Strength and Conditioning Research, 16*(1), 103-108.

Berger, R. (1962). Effect of varied weight training programs on strength. *The Research Quarterly, 33*(2), 169-181.

Boeckh-Behrens, W.-U., & Buskies, W. (2001). *Fitness-Krafttraining [Fitness strength training]* (2nd ed.). Reinbek bei Hamburg: Rowohlt.

Bortz, J., & Lienert, G. A. (2003). *Kurzgefasste Statistik für die klinische Forschung [Statistics for clinical research]* (2nd ed.). Berlin: Springer.

Dons, B., Bollerup, K., Bonde-Petersen, F., & Hancke, S. (1979). The effect of weight-lifting exercise related to muscle fiber composition and muscle cross-sectional area in humans. *European Journal of Applied Physiology and Occupational Physiology, 40*(2), 95-106.

Ebben, W. P., & Blackard, D. O. (2001). Strength and conditioning practices of national football league strength and conditioning coaches. *Journal of Strength and Conditioning Research, 15*(1), 48-58.

Feigenbaum, M. S., & Pollock, M. J. (1997). Strength training. *The Physician and Sportsmedicine, 25*(2), 44-64.

Fleck, S. J., & Kraemer, W. J. (2004). *Designing resistance training programs* (3rd ed.). Champaign, IL: Human Kinetics.

Gießing, J. (2005). Intensive Nachermüdung als Maßnahme zur Optimierung der Ausbelastungsintensität beim Muskelaufbautraining [Post-exhaustion method to optimize intensity of exertion in muscular hypertrophy training]. *Leistungssport, 35*(2), 11-14.

Hass, C. J., Garzarella, L., de Hoyos, D., & Pollock, M. L. (2000). Single versus multiple sets in long-term recreational weightlifters. *Medicine & Science in Sports & Exercise, 32*(1), 235-242.

Heiduk, R., Preuss, P., & Steinhöfer, D. (2002). Die optimale Satzzahl im Krafttraining: Einsatz- versus Mehrsatz-Training [The optimal number of sets: single-set versus multiple-set training]. *Leistungssport, 32*(4), 4-13.

Herm, K.-P. (2003). Methoden der Körperfettbestimmung [Assessment of body composition]. *Deutsche Zeitschrift für Sportmedizin, 54*(5), 153-154.

Hollmann, W., Hettinger, T., & Strüder, H. (2000). *Sportmedizin - Grundlagen für Arbeit, Training und Präventivmedizin [Sports medicine - fundamentals of labour, training and prevention medicine]* (4th ed.). Stuttgart, New York: Schattauer.

Jacobson, B. H. (1986). A comparison of two progressive weight training techniques on knee extensor strength. *Athletic Training, 21*(4), 315-318, 390.

Kraemer, W. J. (1997). A series of studies-the physiological basis for strength training in american football: fact over philosophy. *Journal of Strength and Conditioning Research, 11*(3), 131-142.

Kraemer, W. J., & Häkkinen, K. (Eds.) (2002). *Strength training for sport*. Oxford: Blackwell Science.

Kramer, J. B., Stone, M. H., O'Bryant, H. S., Conley, M. S., Johnson, R. L., Niemann, D. C., et al. (1997). Effects of single vs. multiple sets of weight training: impact of volume, intensity and variation. *Journal of Strength and Conditioning Research, 11*(3), 143-147.

Marx, J. O., Ratamess, N. A., Nindl, B. C., Gotshalk, L. A., Volek, J. S., Dohi, K., et al. (2001). Low-volume circuit versus high-volume periodized resistance training in women. *Medicine & Science in Sports & Exercise, 33*(4), 635-643.

Paulsen, G., Myklestad, D., & Raastad, T. (2003). The influence of volume of exercise on early adaptations to strength training. *Journal of Strength and Conditioning Research, 17*(1), 115-120.

Pollock, M. L., Garzarella, L., & Graves, J. E. (1995). The measurement of body composition. In P. J. Maud & C. Foster, *Physiological assessment of human fitness* (pp. 167-204). Champaign, IL: Human Kinetics.

Rhea, M. R., Alvar, B. A., Ball, S. D., & Burkett, L. N. (2002). Three sets of weight training superior to 1 set with equal intensity for eliciting strength. *Journal of Strength and Conditioning Research, 16*(4), 525-529.

Rhea, M. R., Alvar, B. A., Burkett, L. N., & Ball, S. D. (2003). A meta-analysis to determine the dose response for strength development. *Medicine & Science in Sports & Exercise, 35*(3), 456-464.

Sachs, L. (2002). *Angewandte Statistik [Applied statistic]* (10th ed.). Berlin: Springer.

Sanborn, K., Boros, R., Hruby, J., Schilling, B., O'Bryant, H. S., Johnson, R. L., et al. (2000). Short-term performance effects of weight training with multiple sets not to failure vs. a single set to failure in women. *Journal of Strength and Conditioning Research, 14*(3), 328-331.

Schlumberger, A., & Schmidtbleicher, D. (1999). Einsatz-Training als trainingsmethodische Alternative - Möglichkeiten und Grenzen [Single-set training as methodical alternative - potentials and limits]. *Leistungssport, 29*(3), 9-11

Schlumberger, A., Stec, J., & Schmidtbleicher, D. (2001). Single- vs. multiple-set strength training in women. *Journal of Strength and Conditioning Research, 15*(3), 284-289.

Starkey, D. B., Pollock, M. L., Ishida, Y., Welsch, M. A., Brechue, W. F., Graves, J. E., et al. (1996). Effect of resistance training volume on strength and muscle thickness. *Medicine & Science in Sports & Exercise, 28*(10), 1311-1320.

Stowers, T. (1983). The short term effects of three differnet strength-power training methods. *National Strength and Conditioning Association Journal, 5*(3), 24-27.

Weingarten, B. A. (2000). Bodybuilding HIT. In M. Brzycki, *Maximize your training : insights from leading strength and fitness professionals* (pp. 319-334). Lincolnwood, IL: Masters Press.

Wolfe, B. L., LeMura, L. M., & Cole, P. J. (2004). Quantitative analysis of single- vs. multiple-set programs in resistance training. *Journal of Strength and Conditioning Research, 18*(1), 35-47.

JÜRGEN GIEßING, PETER PREUSS & MICHAEL FRÖHLICH

High-intensity post-exhaustion for maximizing training intensity in muscle hypertrophy training

Keywords: high-intensity training methods, exhaustion, hypertrophy, muscle size, strength

Introduction

It is generally accepted that using repetition maximums (RM), i.e. realizing the maximum number of repetitions that can be accomplished with a certain resistance, is beneficial for inducing muscular hypertrophy (Greiwing, Freiwald, & Nolten, 2003; Heiduk, Preuss, & Steinhöfer, 2002; Philipp, 1999a). Although some authors do not agree with this (Hatfield, 1984; Stone et al., 1998), taking sets to the point of momentary muscular failure (PMF) or even beyond has been found to be very efficient for improving muscle size and strength (Bührle & Werner, 1984; Heiduk et al., 2002; Philipp, 1999a, 1999b; Zatsiorsky, 1996). The point of momentary failure (PMF) is defined as the moment when it becomes impossible to complete the last repetition of a set without compromising good form or having a training partner help the athlete finishing that repetition.
Hatfield (1984) points out that muscular hypertrophy can also be induced without going to failure. According to Hatfield training intensity has to reach a certain threshold in order to stimulate muscular growth.
The argument that muscle growth can also realized without going to failure is undoubtedly true and none of the authors mentioned above disagrees with this notion. However, it has been shown repeatedly that by training to failure muscle gains can be achieved which are superior to those induced by terminating sets before the failure has been reached (Bührle & Werner, 1984; Greiwing et al., 2003; Heiduk et al., 2002; Philipp, 1999a; Rooney, Herbert, & Balnave, 1994). Stone et al. (1998, p. 24) do not agree with the concept of training to failure:

> "The rational for training to failure is that during a set of resistance training exercise, as some motor units fatique and drop out, other motor units must be recruited for continued activity. Fatique allows additional motor units to be trained so the resulting gains in hypertrophy and strength are greater. If fatigue and exercise to failure were the critical factor for enhancing strength, rate of force development, power etc., then one should simply be able to exercise to failure with very light resistances and produce marked gains in hypertrophy and maximum

> strength. But in practice it quickly becomes obvious that this method would not be very efficient in providing an appropriate stimulus for hypertrophy or strength gains."

In this interpretation by Stone et al. (1998) it is not taken into consideration that simply exercising "to failure with very light resistances" will result in fatigue, too, but can not be compared to training to failure for enhancing muscular size and strength: Exercising "with very light resistances" means that a low relative intensity is applied whereas training to failure for increasing muscle size and strength requires medium to high relative intensities.

Although several studies have confirmed that training to muscular failure does effectively stimulate muscular growth and strength increases, this aspect can not be discussed without taking into consideration that training volume is another factor which contributes to muscular failure. The question whether single-set training may produce similar or even superior adaptation is still being discussed (Carpinelli & Otto, 1998; De Hoyos et al., 1997; Feigenbaum & Pollock, 1997; Gießing, 2000, 2002, 2004; Hass, Garzarella, De Hoyos, & Pollock, 1998; Hass, Garzarella, de Hoyos, & Pollock, 2000; Heiduk et al., 2002; Kieser, 1998; Kramer et al., 1997; Marx et al., 1998; Messier & Dill, 1985; Philipp, 1999a, 1999b; Pollock, 1998; Sanborn et al., 1998; Schlumberger & Schmidtbleicher, 1999; Schlumberger, Stec, & Schmidtbleicher, 2001; Starkey et al., 1996; Stone et al., 1998).

Training methods for training to failure and beyond

In order to train to the point of momentary muscular failure (PMF) or even beyond several "high-intensity training methods" (HITM) have been developed and are often applied in strength training in general and in bodybuilding in particular. These HITM were developed and applied by bodybuilders because of empirical evidence that high training intensities very effectively induce increases in muscle size and strength.

Cheating

One of the first HITM was "cheating" which was described as early as 1954 in the bodybuilding magazine muscle builder (Weider, 1954, pp. 60f.). After doing as many repetitions as possible in strict form, athletes are then supposed to "cheat" by using momentum in order to finish some additional repetitions. The effectiveness of this HITM depends very much on its proper application. If athletes cheat to soon or too much, this will inevitably result in a reduction of training intensity rather than in an increase. Improper use of cheating may also "increase the chance of injury" (Fleck & Kraemer, 2004, p. 196). Therefore cheating should always be done carefully and should only be used after the PMF has been reached using very strict form. A major advantage of this HITM is that can be applied without the use of a training partner.

Forced repetitions

After the PMF has been reached, a trainee completes a few additional repetitions with a training partner helping just enough for the repetitions to be completed (Bührle & Werner, 1984).

Partial repetitions

Partial repetitions as a way to increase the training intensity of a set were first described by Richford (1966). If the PMF has been reached and the trainee is too fatigued to finish additional repetitions over the full range of motion, he or she might still be able to do some more partial repetitions. Apart from the fact that this HITM, too, can be applied without the help of a training partner, the main advantage of this HITM is that in contrast to cheating there is no need to compromise good form.

Drop sets

This HITM can also be applied without the help of a training partner. After the PMF has been reached, the weight is reduced by ten to 30 percent so that additional repetitions can be completed. When training with a barbell, weights are "stripped off" both sides of the barbell, which is why this HITM is also called "stripping". If dumbells are used, it is called "working down the rack" because after the maximum number of repetitions has been done, the dumbells are re-racked and a lighter set of dumbells is taken. This way the trainee works his way "down the rack."

Compound sets/super sets

A super set is a combination of two sets that are performed without resting after the first set. The break between the first and the second set of the superset is only as long as it takes to move on from one exercise to the next. If both exercises of the superset are performed for the same muscle group (e.g. preacher-curls and standing barbell curls for the biceps), it is called a superset.

If exercises are chosen which train antagonistic muscles (e.g. biceps curls and triceps extensions), it is called a compound set.

Pre-exhaustion

A special way of performing compound sets is combining a single-joint exercise like leg extensions and a multiple-joint exercise like squats. Pre-exhaustion was first described by Darden (1983). A typical example of pre-exhaustion is performing bench presses immediately after doing a set of dumbell flies to failure. Pre-exhaustion training is based on the assumption that large muscles like the chest can not be trained effectively by doing multiple-joint exercises like bench presses because of the relative weakness of the smaller muscles like the triceps which also contract during the execution of the bench press. It is assumed that the smaller muscles will fatigue before the target muscle (in this example the pectoralis muscles) could be trained to failure. Therefore, single-joint exercises like dumbell flies are done in order to pre-exhaust the pectoralis muscles without exhausting the triceps, so that during the following set of bench presses the triceps are relatively stronger than without pre-exhaustion.

The effectiveness of pre-exhaustion

In order to find out whether pre-exhaustion does indeed create the desired effect, Augustsson et al. (2003) had 17 male subjects do one set of leg presses immediately after performing a set of leg extensions. All subjects were experienced weight trainers who had been training for several years on a recreational level. Leg extensions as well as leg presses were taken to failure using loads that represented 10-RM. The results of this study show that the effectiveness of pre-exhaustion training has not only been vastly overestimated but actually resulted in a decreased activation of the target muscle:

> "Our study showed that pre-exhaustion exercise had the exact opposite effect on muscle activation as suggested by weight trainers using this technique. In our study, pre-exhaustion exercise (a single joint knee extension exercise) resulted in decreased, rather than increased, activation of the quadriceps muscle during a multijoint leg press exercise. Subjects also performed less repetitions of the leg press exercise when in a pre-exhausted state. Thus the lower muscle activity and reduction of strength when using pre-exhaustion exercise compared with regular weight training implies the pre-exhaustion technique may be less effective in muscle development and strength acquisition." (Augustsson et al., 2003, p. 414)

The authors suggest that doing supersets which consist of exercises which train antagonistic muscles might be more effective. In a study by Maynard and

Ebben (2003) the kind of antagonistic pre-exhaustion suggested by Augustsson et al. (2003) was examined. Maynard and Ebben (2003) had 20 male subjects who were also experienced weight trainers perform a set of leg extensions at 5-RM either with or without having done a set of leg curls immediately before. There was no increase in EMG-activity of the m. quadriceps femoris when leg extensions were performed after leg curls. What the authors did find, however, was a significant reduction in strength levels after antagonistic pre-exhaustion:

> "In other words, prefatiguing the antagonist appears to be most detrimental to torque output of the quadriceps (...) and suggests a limitation to agonist-antagonist superset training." (Maynard & Ebben, 2003, p. 469)

Post-exhaustion

Since pre-exhaustion has been found to be less effective than it was previously thought to be, alternative ways of increasing the effectiveness of multiple-joint exercises have to be found. One way of increasing training intensity in the target muscle (groups) when performing multiple-joint exercises is post-exhaustion. Although pre-exhaustion does not necessarily result in the desired effect, there is no doubt that the effectiveness of doing multiple-joint exercises for larger muscles like the m. pectoralis is reduced by the relative weakness of smaller muscles like the triceps that also contract during the execution of multiple-joint exercises like the bench press. If the smaller muscles are already fatigued, the larger muscles cannot be trained with adequate intensity as shown by Sforzo and Tuoey (1996).

Since pre-exhaustion does not provide a solution for this problem, the logical consequence of these findings can only be reversing the order of the exercises performed. Since it is true that the relative weakness of smaller muscles affects training intensity negatively when performing multiple-joint exercises, it is obvious that multiple-joint exercises should be performed first. After the set has been taken to the PMF, it is immediately followed by a single-joint exercise which does not depend on the strength of the smaller muscles as much as the execution of a multiple-joint exercise does. A list of supersets for post-exhaustion is shown in table 1.

Table 1: Post-exhaustion super sets

target muscle	super set consisting of	
	1. a multiple-joint exercise	2. a single-joint exercise
m. pectoralis	bench presses	cable crossovers
m. latissimus	chin-ups to the neck, shoulder-wide grip	dumbell pullovers
m. quadrizeps	leg presses	leg extensions
m. ischiocrurales	stiff-legged deadlift	leg curls
m. deltoideus	front presses	lateral raises
m. trapezius	upright rows	shruggs
m. glutaeus maximus	deadlift	good mornings
Both exercises are taken to failure within 6-RM to 12-RM. The breaks between sets should not exceed 30 seconds.		

High-intensity post-exhaustion

Another advantage of post-exhaustion is that it allows the application of additional HITM like drop sets or forced repetitions. When performing traditional pre-exhaustion adding more HITM would not be recommended since this would add to the undesired effect of making the smaller muscles fatigue even more. If a set of leg extensions done prior to a set of squats results in a reduced EMG-activity in the m. quadriceps, it does not make any sense to add forced repetitions or other HITM to the set of leg extensions because this would make this discrepancy even worse. Using post-exhaustion in order to increase training intensity, however, this is not a problem since the supersets always begin with the multiple-joint exercise. Therefore, training intensity can be increased tremendously by adding HITM like forced repetitions or drop sets to the multiple-joint exercises and then moving on to the single-joint exercise. Very advanced athletes might even go one step further and add forced repetitions or drop set to the single-joint exercise which follows the multiple-set exercise (table 2).

Table 2: High-intensity post-exhaustion

target muscle	super set consisting of:	
	1. a multiple-joint exercise	2. a single-joint exercise
m. pectoralis	bench presses, PMF (or RM if no spotter is available) plus 2 or 3 forced repetitions	cable crossovers PMF plus 1 drop set
m. latissimus	chin-ups to the neck, shoulder-wide grip, PMF plus 4 or 5 partial repetitions	dumbell pullovers, PMF plus 1 drop set
m. quadrizeps	leg presses RM plus 1 drop set	leg extensions PMF plus 1 drop set
mm. ischiocrurales	stiff-legged deadlift RM plus 1 drop set	leg curls PMF plus 1 drop set
m. deltoideus	front presses PMF plus 1 drop set	lateral raises PMF plus 1 drop set
m. trapezius	upright rows PMF plus 4 or 5 partial repetitions	shruggs PMF plus 1 drop set
m. glutaeus maximus	deadlift RM plus 1 drop set	good mornings RM plus 1 drop set
Since additional HITMs are applied here, the TUT should be kept in an optimal range by reaching failure within 5-RM to 8-RM, then the set is continued by applying the HITMs shown in this table. When doing exercises like deadlifts or good mornings it is not advised to train to failure for safety reasons. Therefore, an RM should be performed on these exercises rather than going to the PMF. Trainees who apply HITMs in their workouts should not train without a spotter because when reaching the PMF it can become difficult to control the weight. It is also essential to use proper form for all exercises.		

Conclusion

It has been shown many times that taking a set to the PMF or even beyond is a very effective way to induce increases in muscle size and strength. The results of the research cited above demonstrate that not all methods that are applied in order to increase training intensity are equally effective for that purpose.

Whereas most trainees and coaches are well aware of the disadvantages of several HITMs like e. g. cheating, recent studies show that pre-exhaustion has also been overestimated. This could be shown for regular pre-exhaustion as well as for antagonistic pre-exhaustion. Nevertheless, the combination of a multiple-joint exercise and a single-joint exercise must be considered a very effective way of avoiding the so-called weak links. By reversing the order of exercises the problems described above can be avoided. Another advantage of using post-exhaustion instead of pre-exhaustion is that additional HITMs can be applied, which offers a very efficient way of training beyond the PMF.

References

Augustsson, J., Thomee, R., Hornstedt, P., Lindblom, J., Karlsson, J., & Grimby, G. (2003). Effect of pre-exhaustion exercise on lower-extremity muscle activation during a leg press exercise. *Journal of Strength and Conditioning Research, 17*(2), 411-416.

Bührle, M., & Werner, E. (1984). Das Muskelquerschnittstraining der Bodybuilder [Muscle-hypertrophy training by bodybuilders]. *Leistungssport, 14*(3), 5-9.

Carpinelli, R. N., & Otto, R. M. (1998). Strength training. Single versus multiple sets. *Sports Medicine, 26*(2), 73-84.

Darden, E. (1983). The pre-exhaustion principle in strength training. *Athletic Journal, 1*(46), 66-67.

De Hoyos, D., Herring, D., Garzarella, L., Werber, G., Brechue, W. F., & Pollock, M. L. (1997). Effect of strength training volume on the development of strength and power in adolescent tennis players. *Medicine & Science in Sports & Exercise, 30*(5), S164.

Feigenbaum, M. S., & Pollock, M. L. (1997). Strength training - rationale for current guidelines for adult fitness programs. *Physician and Sports Medicine, 25*(2), 44-46, 49, 54-56, 63, 64.

Fleck, S. J., & Kraemer, W. J. (2004). *Designing resistance training programs* (3rd ed.). Champaign, IL: Human Kinetics.

Gießing, J. (2000). Das Heavy-Duty-Konzept. Zunehmende Akzeptanz und Popularität des Einsatz-Trainings auch beim Bodybuilding [The Heavy-Duty-Concept. Increasing acceptance and popularity of single-set training in bodybuilding]. *Leistungssport, 30*(4), 19-23.

Gießing, J. (2002). *Das Muskelaufbautraining der Bodybuilder. Eine kritische Analyse aus sportwissenschaftlicher Sicht [The hypertrophy training complex used in bodybuilding - a critical analysis from a sport scientific perspective]*. Marburg: Tectum Verlag.

Gießing, J. (2004). *1 Satz Training - Ein wissenschaftlich fundiertes Konzept für schnellstmöglichen Muskelaufbau im Bodybuilding [Single-set training. A concept for rapid muscle gains based on scientific findings]* (1st ed.). Arnsberg: Novagenics.

Greiwing, A., Freiwald, J., & Nolten, J. (2003). Der Einfluss zweier Krafttrainingsmethoden mit dem "Kettler Multitrainer" auf isometrische Maximalkraft und Befindlichkeit [The influence of two different strength training methods with the "Kettler-Mulititrainer" on maximum isometric strength and existential orientation]. *Gesundheitssport und Sporttherapie, 19*, 208-213.

Hass, C. J., Garzarella, L., De Hoyos, D., & Pollock, M. L. (1998). Effects of training volume on strength and endurance in experienced resistance trained adults. *Medicine & Science in Sports & Exercise, 30*(5), 208-214.

Hass, C. J., Garzarella, L., de Hoyos, D., & Pollock, M. L. (2000). Single versus multiple sets in long-term recreational weightlifters. *Medicine & Science in Sports & Exercise, 32*(1), 235-242.

Hatfield, F. (1984). *Bodybuilding - A Scientific Approach*. Chicago, IL: Contemporary Books.

Heiduk, R., Preuss, P., & Steinhöfer, D. (2002). Die optimale Satzzahl im Krafttraining: Einsatz- versus Mehrsatz-Training [The optimal number of sets: single-set versus multiple-set training]. *Leistungssport, 32*(4), 4-13.

Kieser, W. (1998). Wieviele Sätze beim Krafttraining? Theorie und Praxis [How much sets in strength training? Theory and practice]. *Leistungssport, 28*(3), 50-51.

Kramer, J. B., Stone, M. H., O'Bryant, H. S., Conley, M. S., Johnson, R. L., Nieman, D. C., et al. (1997). Effects of single vs. multiple sets of weight training: impact of volume, intensity, and variation. *Journal of Strength and Conditioning Research, 11*(3), 143-147.

Marx, J. O., Nindl, B. C., Gothshalk, L. A., Volek, J. S., Harmann, F. S., Dohi, K., et al. (1998). The effects of a low-volume progressive resistance exercise program versus a high-volume periodized resistance exercise program on muscular performance in women. In K. Häkkinen (Ed.), *International conference on weightlifting and strength training* (pp. 167-168). Lathi, Finland: Gummerus Printing.

Maynard, J., & Ebben, W. P. (2003). The effects of antagonist prefatigue on agonist torque and electromyography. *Journal of Strength and Conditioning Research, 17*(3), 469-474.

Messier, S. P., & Dill, M. E. (1985). Alterations in strength and maximal oxygen uptake consequent to Nautilus circuit weight training. *Research Quarterly for Exercise and Sport, 56*(4), 345-351.

Philipp, M. (1999a). Ein Satz genügt! - Erfahrungen mit Mehrsatz- und Einsatz-Methoden im Krafttraining. Eine Fallstudie als Diskussionsbeitrag zur Anregung von Werner Kieser [One set is enough! - Experiences with multilpe-set and single-set training in strength training. A case study to adress the controversy with Werner Kieser]. *Leistungssport, 29*(1), 26-28.

Philipp, M. (1999b). Einsatz-Training versus Mehrsatz-Training. Zur Kontroverse um die Satzzahl beim Krafttraining unter Berücksichtigung empirischer Evidenzen [Single-set versus multiple-set training. To adress the controversy under consideration of empirical data]. *Leistungssport, 29*(4), 27-34.

Pollock, M. L. (1998). Muscular hypertrophy responses to 6 months of high- or low-volume resistance training. *Medicine & Science in Sports & Exercise, 30*(5), S116.

Richford, C. (1966). *Principles of successful bodybuilding*: Alliance.

Rooney, K. J., Herbert, R. D., & Balnave, R. J. (1994). Fatigue contributes to the strength training stimulus. *Medicine & Science in Sports & Exercise, 26*(9), 1160-1164.

Sanborn, K., Boros, R., Hruby, J., Schilling, B., O´Bryant, H., Johnson, R., et al. (1998). Performance effecte of weigth training with multiple sets not to failure versus a single set to failure in women: a prelimenary study. In K. Häkkinen (Ed.), *International conference on weigthlifting and strength training* (pp. 157-158). Lathi, Finnland: Gummerus Printing.

Schlumberger, A., & Schmidtbleicher, D. (1999). Einsatz-Training als trainingsmethodische Alternative - Möglichkeiten und Grenzen [Single-set training as methodical alternative - potentials and limits]. *Leistungssport, 29*(3), 9-11.

Schlumberger, A., Stec, J., & Schmidtbleicher, D. (2001). Single- vs. multiple-set strength training in women. *Journal of Strength and Conditioning Research, 15*(3), 284-289.

Sforzo, G. A., & Touey, P. R. (1996). Manipulating exercise order affects muscular performance during a resistance exercise training session. *Journal of Strength and Conditioning Research, 10*(1), 20-24.

Starkey, D. B., Pollock, M. L., Ishida, Y., Welsch, M. A., Brechue, W. F., Graves, J. E., et al. (1996). Effect of resistance training volume on strength and muscle thickness. *Medicine & Science in Sports & Exercise, 28*(10), 1311-1320.

Stone, M. H., Plisk, S. S., Stone, M. E., Schilling, B. K., O´Bryant, H. S., & Pierce, K. C. (1998). Athletic performance development: Volume load-1 set vs. multiple sets, training velocity and training variation. *Strength and Conditioning Journal, 20*(6), 22-31.

Weider, J. (1954). Cheating exercise build the biggest muscles. *Muscle Builder, 3*, 60-61.

Zatsiorsky, V. M. (1996). *Krafttraining - Wissenschaft und Praxis [Science and practice of strength training]*. Aachen: Meyer & Meyer.

HUBERT REMMERT, ALEXANDER SCHISCHEK, TOBIAS ZAMHÖFER &
ALEXANDER FERRAUTI

Influence of recovery duration on increase of strength and muscular growth within a high-intensity training (HIT)

Keywords: muscular growth, high-intensity training, single-set training, training volume, time under tension

Introduction

The pros and cons of low-volume training (LVT) as a methodological alternative to classic high-volume training (HVT) have recently been discussed very actively in German literature (e.g. Gießing, 2000; Gießing, 2002; Kieser, 1998; Philipp, 1999a, 1999b; Schlumberger & Schmidtbleicher, 1999). At the same time, research concerning possible preferences of low or high-volume training concepts regarding training effects can only be denominated as unclear (Dachilau, Stein, Schäfer, Buhlmann, & Menken, 2004). This is even more astonishing as arguments concerning LVT or HVT are partly being presented rather dogmatically (Szubski, 1999). Besides, the vague definitional classification of LVT - usually an essential prerequisite for methodological criticism and comparison - comes as a surprise. Anyhow, it appears to be clear that there have to be made distinctions between specific training methods within the organisational form of LVT. Their selection and efficiency are determined by concrete training objectives and initial conditions - what has been a matter of course in the field of HVT for decades. As to this, Heiduk, Preuss and Steinhöfer (2002) differentiate low-volume training methods according to choice of exercise and criteria of strain. Their suggestion will be complemented by us with the so called body building single-set training (B-SST) (figure 1).

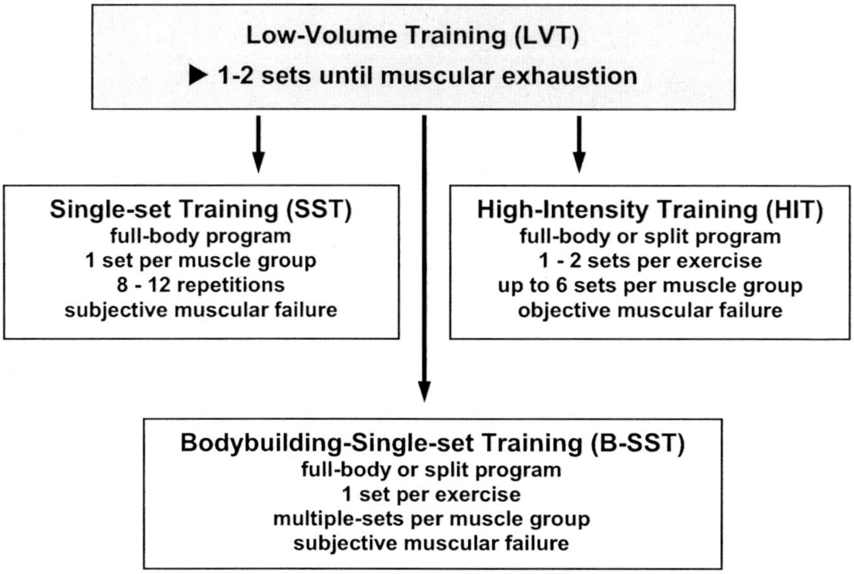

Figure 1: Low-volume training methods (cf. Heiduk et al., 2002; Schischek & Zamhöfer, 2004)

The LVT-specific method of high-intensity training (HIT) is characterized by its objective strain on the trained muscular system within only one set of each exercise. This is achieved by a particularly slow exercise of movement and the application of different resistance training techniques (e.g. breakdown sets) in subsequent connection to the concentric muscular failure (subjective strain). It is being assumed that the resultant profound exhaustion of the confluence of bodily energy leads to an enhanced activation of protein synthesis and muscular growth (e.g. Brzycki, 1995; Gießing, 2002; Hemmling, 1994; Kieser, 1998; Stone, Chandler, Conley, Kramer, & Stone, 1996; Zatsiorsky, 1992). A HIT can be characterized as follows:

a) one set per exercise,
b) slow and controlled repetition speed (2 s concentric, 1 s isometric, 4 s eccentric),
c) objective strain of the stressed muscular groups by techniques of intensity (HITM) subsequent to concentric muscular failure.

Within the scope of their study Heiduk et al. (2002) were able to prove the extraordinary efficiency of a HIT for weight and strength trained athletes (cp. Müller, 2003; Szubski, 1999). The question that remained to be clarified was that of the ideal proportionality between strain and recreation in the context of this highly demanding workout which even as a three-day split caused overtraining symptoms (e.g. severe and persistent exhaustion, loss of motivation and recessive performance, cp. Heiduk et al., 2002). In this current study we take up this unanswered question - which is fundamental for the concrete monitoring of training - and look into the impact of different recreation intervals on adaptation effects with regards to strength and muscular circumference development during a full-body HIT.

Methodology

Two randomised groups each consisting of ten male athletes experienced in weight training did an identical full-body training regimen (table 1) according to the strain components of a HIT for twelve weeks. Apart from the facultative abdominal workout the training exercises were performed on gym equipment in order to guarantee injury prevention.

Group 1 (G1: age 30.4 ± 7.3 years, weight 89.0 ± 18.0 kg, height 1.82 ± 0.1 m, BMI 26.8 ± 4.2) worked out once a week with approximately 166 hours of recreation and consequently completed a total training work load of 12 training units during the testing period.

Group 2 (G2: age 30.0 ± 8.0 years, weight 78.9 ± 10.6 kg, height 1.79 ± 0.1 m, BMI 24.5 ± 2.7) completed two units per week with recreation intervals of 70 or 94 hours. So members of group 2 did a whole work load of 24 training units (figure 2). The subjects were not permitted further training during the testing period. Miscellaneous sportive activities were recorded. Significant differences between the two training groups could not be detected.

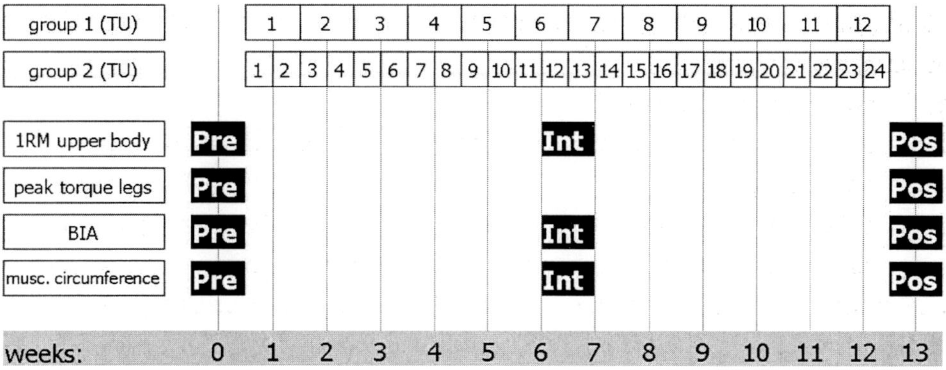

Figure 2: Investigational design (Pre = pre-test, Int = intermediate test, Post = post-test

Table 1: Training regimen of a full-body HIT during the training period

sequence	exercise	time under tension	breakdown sets
E 1	leg press	60 - 90 s	1 + 1
E 2	leg extension	60 - 90 s	1 + 1
E 3	harmstring curl	60 - 90 s	1 + 1
E 4	calf raise	60 - 90 s	1 + 1
E 5	back extension	60 - 90 s	-
E 6	pull-over	40 - 70 s	1 + 1
E 7	latissimus pull-down	40 - 70 s	1 + 1
E 8	biceps curls	40 - 70 s	1 + 1
E 9	arm fly	40 - 70 s	1 + 1
E 10	bench press	40 - 70 s	1 + 1
E 11	triceps press-down	40 - 70 s	1 + 1
E 12	shoulder raise	40 - 70 s	1 + 1
optional	abdominal workout (sit-ups, side-ups, straight-ups)	subjective strain	-

Monitoring of training was accomplished by time under tension (TUT). First-time muscular failure was to occur during concentric leg exercises between 60 and 90 seconds, during upper body exercises between 40 and 70 seconds (Castellano, 2000; Kieser, 2000; Platonov, 1999). This was followed by two breakdown sets leaving out exercise 5 (E5, back extension) and the abdominal workout. The machine's weight was reduced for two plates during the first and for one more plate during the second reduced set. Resting periods between workout exercises were 2:30 minutes each.

If the weight could be moved beyond the maximum time of tension until concentric muscular failure occurred more weight was added. In case of failing the minimum the weight was reduced accordingly (figure 3).

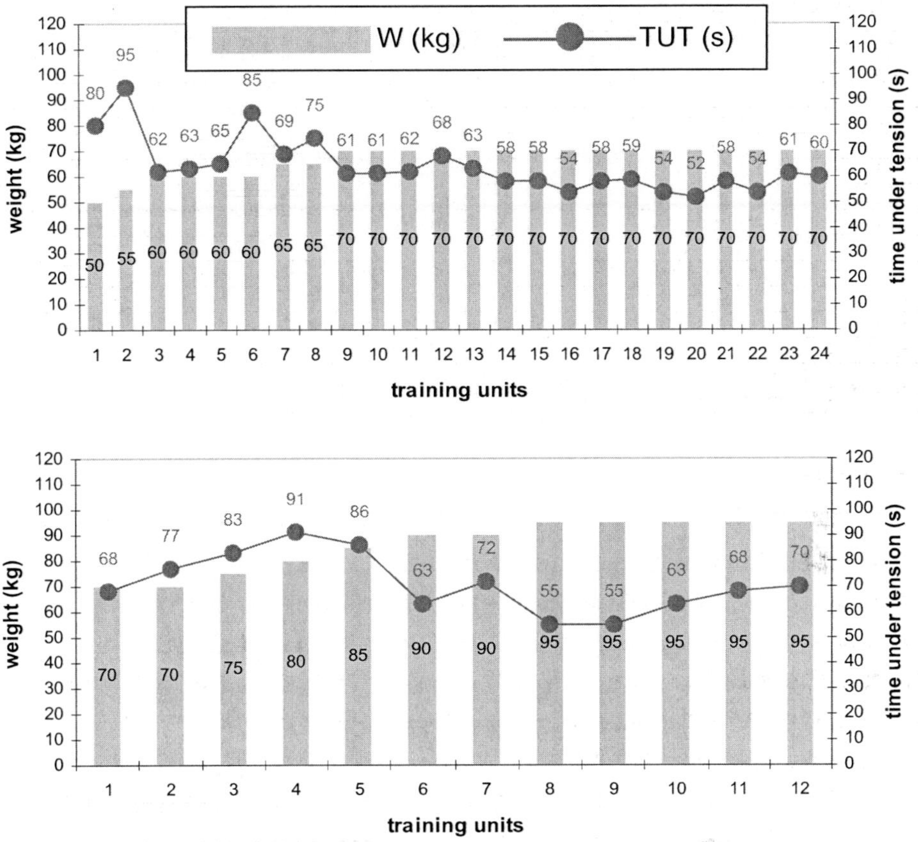

Figure 3: Alteration of time under tension (TUT) and training weight (W) over the total period shown by the example of pullover exercise of two subjects of G1 (1 TU/week) and G2 (2TU/week)

During pre-, intermediate and post-tests (Pre, Int, Post) measurements of maximum force production have been carried out employing 1-RM seated bench press and 1-RM latissimus pull-down as well as isokinetic measurements of force regarding knee extensors and flexors (these Pre and Post only). Furthermore, data concerning potential effects of muscle hypertrophy (bioelectrical impedance analysis - BIA, circumference measuring) were collected (figure 2; table 2).

*Table 2: Testing procedures and time of testing, *1-RM (Heiduk et al., 2002)*

	Pre	Int	Post
1-RM* seated bench press, upright position (training equipment of GYM 80, Gelsenkirchen, G)	X	X	X
1-RM* latissimus pull-down, fixation of the thighs (training equipment of GYM, Gelsenkirchen, G)	X	X	X
peak torque of knee extensors at 60°/s (KINTREX 1000, Meditronic Instruments, Ecublens, CH)	X	-	X
peak torque of knee flexors at 60°/s (KINTREX 1000, Meditronic Instruments, Ecublens, CH)	X	-	X
muscular quantity after 4-point-bioelectrical impedance analysis (BIACOM, software BIAWIN 3.2)	X	X	X
upper arm circumference in cm, right-angled flexion of elbow joint with horizontally upraised arm and max. contraction of elbow flexors (according to Tittel & Wutscherk, 1972)	X	X	X
thighs circumference in cm, 20 cm proximal to lateral knee joint gap at max. contraction in upstanding position (according to Tittel & Wutscherk, 1972)	X	X	X

Statistical procedure

Statistical analysis of the ascertained values was utilized descriptically and analytically (Software SPSS 11.5) by means of analysis of variance (ANOVA) with repeated measurements including Levene- and Box-M-test as well as the t-test for independent samples of percentage change analysis between training groups. Statistical significance level was set at $p < 0.05$.

Results

Maximum force tests showed improvements between pre- and post-tests for both of the surveyed training groups (table 3). Also, both groups made continuous progress on the seated bench press from intermediate (G1 +4 kg; G2 +3.7 kg after six weeks) to post-test (G1 +6.5 kg; G2 +6.5 kg after twelve weeks). Measured values of the 1-RM latissimus pull-down show the same development. Peak torque of knee extensors and flexors were also increased at angular velocity of 60 °/s (extensors: G1 +9.5 Nm; G2 +8.4 Nm; flexors: G1 +13.1 Nm; G2 +7.7 Nm).

According to bioelectrical impedance analysis (BIA) the total muscular growth was 0.6 % in G1 and 1.1 % in G2. Moreover, the muscular circumference of the upper arm and thighs developed profitably (upper arm: G1 +0.9 cm; G2 +1.1 cm; thighs: G1 + 1.9 cm; G2 +1.3cm). The BIA as well as circumference measuring resulted in positive increase during the first (pre- to intermediate test) and the second (intermediate to post-test) half of the training period.

Table 3: Testing results at different points of testing ($\overline{\mathbf{x}} \pm s$)

test item	point of testing	testing group	
		G1 (n = 10; 1 TU/week)	G2 (n = 10; 2 TU/week)
1-RM seated bench press (weight in kg)	PRE	89.5 ± 12.3	87.3 ± 13.2
	INT	93.5 ± 12.2	91.0 ± 15.6
	POST	96.0 ± 11.4	93.8 ± 16.8
1-RM latissimus pull-down (weight in kg)	PRE	87.3 ± 13.8	82.3 ± 6.4
	INT	91.0 ± 14.3	85.3 ± 6.5
	POST	93.8 ± 14.1	88.3 ± 6.4
peak torque of knee extensors (60 °/s, in Nm)	PRE	212.6 ± 48.5	201.8 ± 38.0
	INT	----------	----------
	POST	222.1 ± 49.2	210.2 ± 39.8
peak torque of knee flexors (60 °/s, in Nm)	PRE	147.3 ± 20.8	135.3 ± 21.2
	INT	----------	----------
	POST	160.4 ± 18.7	143.0 ± 21.3
muscle proportion acc. to BIA (in %)	PRE	39.7 ± 3.1	41.1 ± 1.8
	INT	40.1 ± 3.2	41.7 ± 2.1
	POST	40.3 ± 3.0	42.2 ± 2.0
circumference of upper arm (in cm)	PRE	36.7 ± 2.1	35.8 ± 1.8
	INT	37.3 ± 2.1	36.5 ± 2.1
	POST	37.6 ± 2.2	36.9 ± 2.0
circumference of thighs (in cm)	PRE	56.3 ± 5.9	54.3 ± 4.3
	INT	57.0 ± 5.7	54.9 ± 4.8
	POST	58.2 ± 5.1	55.6 ± 4.6

According to analysis of variance (table 4), results show that positive changes between the tests are significant - except for knee extensor and muscular circumference.

The calculated differences can chiefly be explained by inter-subjective effects (time of testing) whereas the percentage of the entire variance come about most obviously at 1-RM seated bench press (72.8 %) and 1-RM latissimus pull-down (84.6 %) (compare η^2). Differences between the two groups cannot be detected. Throughout, the intra-subjective (group) as well as the interactive effects (between time of testing and tested group) do not turn out significantly and percentage-wise do not play a vital role in the clarification of the cumulative variances. Additional t-tests with both the groups (that are not commented on here) did not turn out to be significant.

*Table 4: ANOVA results; * significant ($\alpha = 0.05$)*

test item	ANOVA-effects		
	intra-subjetive (Pillai-Spur)	**inter-subjective**	**interaction (Pillai-Spur)**
1-RM seated bench press	0.000* [$\eta 2 = 0.728$]	0.706 [$\eta 2 = 0.008$]	0.962 [$\eta 2 = 0.005$]
1-RM latissimus pull-down	0.000* [$\eta 2 = 0.846$]	0.279 [$\eta 2 = 0.065$]	0.667 [$\eta 2 = 0.047$]
peak torque of knee extensors	0.065 [$\eta 2 = 0.177$]	0.562 [$\eta 2 = 0.019$]	0.905 [$\eta 2 = 0.001$]
peak torque of knee flexors	0.000* [$\eta 2 = 0.518$]	0.114 [$\eta 2 = 0.133$]	0.268 [$\eta 2 = 0.068$]
muscle proportion (BIA)	0.053 [$\eta 2 = 0.293$]	0.171 [$\eta 2 = 0.101$]	0.650 [$\eta 2 = 0.049$]
upper arm circumference	0.000* [$\eta 2 = 0.702$]	0.374 [$\eta 2 = 0.044$]	0.777 [$\eta 2 = 0.029$]
thighs circumference	0.000* [$\eta 2 = 0.715$]	0.335 [$\eta 2 = 0.052$]	0.378 [$\eta 2 = 0.108$]

Discussion

The key finding of the presented study is that when performing a heavily loaded high-intensity training even extremely long recreational cycles of one week (G1: 1 TU per week) guarantee substantial performance enhancements. Surprisingly, the measured values do not differ statistically from those of the comparable group that performed twice as many training units (G2: 2 TU per week) (figure 5). Apparently, the enormous neuro-muscular exhaustion and possible filamentary destruction induced by a HIT demand generously planned recreational cycles which the organism needs for the rebuilding of the acutely stressed strenght reserves and the damaged contractile proteins (Geiger, 1997; Zatsiorsky, 2000) as well as the neuro-muscular functionality (Ahtiainen, Pakarinen, Kraemer, & Hakkinen, 2003).

Maximum strength parameters of the upper and the lower body significantly and equally improved in both of the tested groups. These positive changes are accompanied by the results of bioelectrical impedance analysis and circumference of upper arms and thighs which, however, in the case of the BIA cannot be statistically substantiated (table 4 and figure 4).

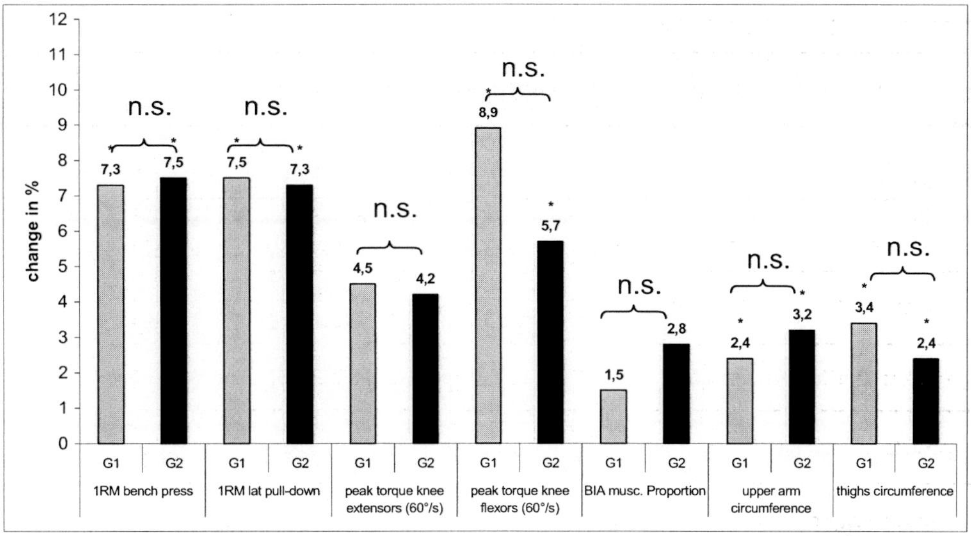

Figure 4: Percentage development of test parameters between pre- and post-test

At the same time we found a tendentially bigger increase of maximum strength at 1-RM seated bench press and 1-RM latissimus pull-down in the first half of the training period (table 3). Due to long-time weight training experience of all subjects coordinative strength increase can largely be ruled out as an explanation. Hypertrophy indicators (BIA and circumference) rather prove a cross-section enlargement already during the first six weeks of the testing period. This exemplifies the remarkably high efficiency of a HIT right after the first six training units (G1: 1TU/week). The tendentially smaller increase in both groups during the second half of the training period seems to indicate that for weight-trained athletes a training program modification in terms of exercise selection and/or training methods have to be made after six to twelve weeks of training (Gießing, 2002, also compare figure 3). Isokinetic strength of lower limbs only improved significantly in part between pre- and post-test. From our point of view this is due to a generally higher initial weekday level primarily of the extensors. The calculated strength increase can chiefly be explained by the coordinative didactic effect regarding the testing procedure the more so as the subjects were inexperienced with the isokinetic measurement process (Dachilau et al., 2004). This corresponds with the result that the amplitude of the thighs tendentially increased stronger not before the second half of the testing period (table 3). Thus, the adjustments of the leg musculature are likely to follow a classic sequence of coordination and hypertrophy.

We consider monitoring of training by time under tension a very practicable way of regulating and documenting training. In combination with the used weight progresses are documented and depicted very precisely (figure 3 and 4). Corresponding with the strength test performances greater progress during the first weeks than during the second half of the study can also be detected here. Yet, towards the end of the study almost stagnation regarding training performances could be detected with most subjects. We think this individual levelling off at a certain performance level is due to the adjustment to the training work load of a HIT which also suggests a modification of the training contents, training methodology and/or training intensity after twelve weeks at the latest or maybe even earlier (see above).
Moreover, an individually precise perfectioning of monitoring of training is subject to manifold factors (genetical predisposition, diet, shape, sleep etc.) that could not be controlled in the context of this study and which consequently make it a must in practice to make out the facts by attempt. Anyhow, it has not been possible to deduce practicable diagnostic routines from sports-medicinal indicators in order to determine optimal recreational cycles for weight training so far. Ascertaining different hormonal (testosterone, cortisol, GH etc.), neuronal (EMG-activity, isometric strength development) and metabolic parameters (blood lactic, creatine kinesis etc.) provided important clues concerning this matter. Due to complex laboratory diagnostics this has not been possible within the limits of this study. Literature points out that due to great central exhaustion effects neuro-muscular functionality is not fully restored even three days after an objective muscular strain - in contrast to a clearly faster recreational process after merely subjective training interventions (Ahtiainen et al., 2003).
Altogether, presented data proves that there still is considerable need for investigating and clarifying resistance training parameters, especially the duration of recovery periods.

Practical training recommendations

Aiming at maximum strength increase and muscular hypertrophy the HIT proves to be a practicable training method. The verifiable efficiency of this variety of Low-volume training makes it an interesting methodological and timesaving alternative to High-volume training. The complete (objective) muscular strain allows a steadily high increased performance even after long recreational periods up to a week between the particular training units.

However, subjective response during the training period showed that G1 subjects contrary to G2 subjects complained of muscular soreness after each training unit. Perhaps active and passive muscular structures need a more frequent training stimulus than once a week in order to establish a functionally tolerance of strain independently of the immediate performance capacity. Accordingly, the optimal recreational period of an entire organism exposed to a HIT depicted as it is here would be between four to six days.

Considering the available results and the personal experiences of the athletes with a HIT we recommend full-body training according to table 5 which combines a HIT and a less exhausting training program on two different days within a seven-day micro-cycle. The second training unit should not lead to complete muscular exhaustion, but follow the recommendations of subjective strain of body-building single-set training (B-SST, see figure 1). This way the necessary functionality of all muscular structures can be sustained without causing overtraining or protein wastage, respectively (Heiduk et al., 2002; Zimmermann, 2000).

Table 5: Hypertrophy-orientated full-body training program for seven days (TUT = time under tension up to muscular failure)

<table>
<tr><th colspan="2">program 1: B-SST day 1</th><th rowspan="6">recreation day 2 - 3</th><th colspan="2">program 2: HIT day 4</th><th rowspan="6">recreation day 5 - 7</th></tr>
<tr><td>leg extension
harmstring curl
calf raise</td><td>TUT 60 - 90 s</td><td>leg press</td><td>TUT 60 - 90 s</td></tr>
<tr><td>dead lift</td><td>TUT 60 - 90 s</td><td>back extension</td><td>TUT 60 - 90 s</td></tr>
<tr><td>arm fly
bench press
triceps press-down</td><td>TUT 40 -70 s</td><td>bench press</td><td>TUT 40 - 70 s</td></tr>
<tr><td>pull-over
latissimus pull-down
biceps curls</td><td>TUT 40 - 70 s</td><td>latissimus pull-down</td><td>TUT 40 - 70 s</td></tr>
<tr><td>shoulder raise</td><td>TUT 40 - 70 s</td><td>shoulder raise</td><td>TUT 40 - 70 s</td></tr>
</table>

The HIT should entirely mind coordinatively demanding, multi-jointed free-handed handling exercises which is due to the increased risk of physical injury at objective strain. Also, they can be deployed during B-SST to modify correlating machine-aided exercises.

In addition to the training suggestion we recommend training of the torso-stabilizing abdominal muscles at least twice a week (e.g. sit-ups, side-ups, straight-ups). This abdominal workout can either be exercised at the end of the two training units or additionally on the days free of training.

References

Ahtiainen, J. P., Pakarinen, A., Kraemer, W. J., & Hakkinen, K. (2003). Acute hormonal and neuromuscular responses and recovery to forced vs maximum repetitions multiple resistance exercises. *International Journal of Sports Medicine, 24*(6), 410-418.

Brzycki, M. (1995). *A practical approach to strength training* (3rd ed.). Lincolnwood, IL: Masters Press.

Castellano, R. (2000). Fibre-types and repetition ranges. In M. Brzycki (Ed.), *Maximize your training: insights from leading strength and fitness professionals* (pp. 213-220). Lincolnwood, IL: Master Press.

Dachilau, S., Stein, B., Schäfer, K., Buhlmann, J. J., & Menken, P. (2004). Einsatz- versus Mehrsatztraining - zwei konkurrierende Krafttrainingsmethoden in der Behandlung chronischer Rückenschmerzen? [Single-set versus multiple-set training - two concurrent strength training methods in the therapy of chronic lower back pain]. *Physikalische Therapie in Theorie und Praxis, 25*(7), 294-299.

Geiger, L. V. (1997). *Überlastungsschäden im Sport [Damages through overstress in sports].* München: BLV Verlag.

Gießing, J. (2000). Das Heavy-Duty-Konzept. Zunehmende Akzeptanz und Popularität des Einsatz-Trainings auch beim Bodybuilding [The Heavy-Duty-Concept. Increasing acceptance and popularity of single-set training in bodybuilding]. *Leistungssport, 30*(4), 19-23.

Gießing, J. (2002). *Das Muskelaufbautraining der Bodybuilder. Eine kritische Analyse aus sportwissenschaftlicher Sicht [The hypertrophy training complex used in bodybuilding - a critical analysis from a sport scientific perspective].* Marburg: Tectum Verlag.

Heiduk, R., Preuss, P., & Steinhöfer, D. (2002). Die optimale Satzzahl im Krafttraining: Einsatz- versus Mehrsatz-Training [The optimal number of sets: single-set versus multiple-set training]. *Leistungssport, 32*(4), 4-13.

Hemmling, G. (1994). *Anpassungen des neuromuskulären Systems an eine neuentwickelte Trainingsmethode [Adaptations of the neuromuscular systems to a newly developed training method].* Köln: Sport und Buch Strauß.

Kieser, W. (1998). Wieviele Sätze beim Krafttraining? Theorie und Praxis [How many sets in strength training? Theory and practice]. *Leistungssport, 28*(3), 50-51.

Kieser, W. (2000). *Ein starker Rücken kennt keinen Schmerz. Gesundheitsorientiertes Krafttraining nach der Kieser-Methode [A strong back knows no pain. Health orientated strength training according to the Kieser-Method].* München: Heyne.

Müller, A. (2003). Zur Transferierbarkeit trainingsmethodischer Erfahrungen des Hochleistungsbodybuildings. Eine kritische Betrachtung des vorliegenden Methodenspektrums [Transferability of methodical knowledge by competitive bodybuilding. A critical reflection of currently methods]. *Leistungssport, 33*(4), 38-42.

Philipp, M. (1999a). Ein Satz genügt! - Erfahrungen mit Mehrsatz- und Einsatz-Methoden im Krafttraining. Eine Fallstudie als Diskussionsbeitrag zur Anregung von Werner Kieser [One set is enough! - Experiences with multilpe-set and single-set training in strength training. A case study to adress the controversy with Werner Kieser]. *Leistungssport, 29*(1), 26-28.

Philipp, M. (1999b). Einsatz-Training versus Mehrsatz-Training. Zur Kontroverse um die Satzzahl beim Krafttraining unter Berücksichtigung empirischer Evidenzen [Single-set versus multiple-set training. To adress the controversy under consideration of empirical data]. *Leistungssport, 29*(4), 27-34.

Platonov, V. N. (1999). *Belastung-Ermüdung-Leistung: Der moderne Trainingsaufbau [Stress-fatigue-performance: the modern planning of training].* Münster: Philippka.

Schischek, A., & Zamhöfer, T. (2004). *Die Auswirkungen eines mehrwöchigen HIT im Hinblick auf die Kraft- und Muskelmassenzunahme mit unterschiedlichen Regenerationszeiten bei fortgeschrittenen Fitness-/Kraftsportlern [The influence of several weeks of high-intensity training on maximum strength and lean body mass increases with different regeneration periods on experienced fitness sportlers].* Unpublished diplomathesis, Ruhr-Universität Bochum, Bochum.

Schlumberger, A., & Schmidtbleicher, D. (1999). Einsatz-Training als trainingsmethodische Alternative - Möglichkeiten und Grenzen [Single-set training as methodical alternative - potentials and limits]. *Leistungssport, 29*(3), 9-11.

Stone, M. H., Chandler, T. J., Conley, M. S., Kramer, J. B., & Stone, M. E. (1996). Training to muscular failure: It is necessary? *Strength and Conditioning, 18*(3), 44-48.

Szubski, C. (1999). Der Einsatz-Training versus Mehrsatz-Training-Dogmatismus - Ein Beispiel für Glaubenslehren in der Trainingswissenschaft? [The single-set versus multiple-set dogmatism - an example for dogma in sport science?]. *Leistungssport, 29*(4), 35.

Tittel, K., & Wutscherk, H. (1972). *Sportanthropometrie [Sportanthropometry].* Leipzig: Johann Ambrosius Barth.

Zatsiorsky, V. M. (1992). Intensity of Strength Training Facts and Theory: Russian and Eastern European Approach. *National Strength and Conditioning Journal, 14*(5), 46-57.

Zatsiorsky, V. M. (2000). *Krafttraining - Wissenschaft und Praxis [Science and practice of strength training]* (2nd ed.). Aachen: Meyer & Meyer.

Zimmermann, K. (2000). *Gesundheitsorientiertes Muskelkrafttraining [Health-orientated strength training].* Schorndorf: Verlag Karl Hofmann.

JÜRGEN GIEßING

Intense single-set training for maximum muscular hypertrophy in bodybuilding

Keywords: single-set training, hypertrophy, multiple-set training, heavy duty, high-intensity

Introduction

A review of the international literature shows that there are reasons to question the necessity of multiple-set training for muscular hypertrophy. The results of recent studies provide proponents of single-set training with several arguments that the importance of strength training volume has been considerably overestimated in the past. The outstanding degree of muscular development achieved by bodybuilders is often used as empirical evidence for the necessity of high training volumes for muscle building:

> "While scientific training studies have typically employed 1 to 4 sets per muscle group per session, elite bodybuilders are reputed to perform from 9 to 24 sets per muscle group in a single training session. Consequently it is generally accepted that high training volumes, say, 3-6 sets per exercise for 3-4 exercises (...) represent the best way to achieve myogenic increases." (Ostrowski, Wilson, Weatherby, Murphy, & Lyttle, 1997, p. 148)

Some authors consider it to be highly unlikely that high-volume training would have become a cornerstone of bodybuilding, if low-volume approaches delivered the same results.

Training methods of bodybuilders

Bodybuilders usually apply a high degree of training intensity and a high training volume. It is common to do several exercises for each muscle group and to do three sets of each exercise. Some authors recommend an even higher volume for muscle building purposes.

Christ (1992) suggests bodybuilders should do up to eight sets per exercise. Fleck/Kraemer (1987, p. 57) even state that there is a direct correlation between training volume and training results:

> "The number of sets used in a workout is directly related to training results."

Koch and Haff (1999, p. 103) consider the volume of a training session to be the key factor for muscular hypertrophy: "A bodybuilding routine produces great gains in muscle size. Most likely, the relatively high volume of sets and reps is the primary reason." Consequently, they recommend a high-volume training schedule (see table 1).

Table 1: Bodybuilding-split-program recommended by Koch and Haff (1999)

first and fourth day	**second and fifth day**	**third and sixth day**
chest, shoulders and triceps	back, biceps and abdominals	thighs and calves
bench press 4 sets of 6 - 10 reps	seated rows 4 sets of 8 - 12 reps	barbell squat 4 sets of 10 - 15 reps
decline bench press 4 sets of 6 - 10 reps	latpulldowns to the back 4 sets of 8 - 12 reps	leg presses 4 sets of 8 - 12 reps
flies 4 sets of 6 - 10 reps	latpulldowns to the front 4 sets of 8 - 12 reps	stiff-legged deadlift 4 sets of 10 - 15 reps
butterfly 4 sets of 6 - 10 reps	dumbbell rows 4 sets of 8 - 12 reps	leg curls 3 sets of 8 - 12 reps
dumbbell frontpress 4 sets of 6 - 10 reps	barbell curl 4 sets of 8 - 12 reps	seated calf raises 4 sets of 8 - 12 reps
lateral dumbbell raises 4 sets of 8 - 12 reps	dumbbell curl 4 sets of 8 - 12 reps	standing calf raises 4 sets of 10 - 15 reps
lateral raises to the back 4 sets of 8 - 12 reps	curls with pronated grip 4 sets of 8 - 12 reps	
triceps extensions 4 sets of 8 - 12 reps	crunch 2-3 sets of 20 - 30 reps	
french press 4 sets of 8 - 12 reps	leg raises 3 sets of 10 - 15 reps	

Another decisive characteristic of bodybuilding training is the application of HITMs that increase training intensity in order to maximally fatigue the target muscle within each training set. It is believed that the degree of fatigue of the trained muscle is an essential factor triggering the stimulation of muscular hypertrophy (Dudley, Tesch, Miller, & Buchanan, 1991; Hemmling, 1994; Jones & Rutherford, 1987). Bührle and Werner (1984) described some of the better-known HITMs like forced reps, partial reps, supersets and pre-exhaustion. Those techniques are called "Weider principles" because they were made popular by bodybuilding magazines and books edited by Joe Weider. However, the term "Weider principles" is misleading in this context since it describes training methods rather than training principles. The goal of all HITMs applied in bodybuilding is to fatigue the trained muscle beyond the "point of momentary muscular failure" (PMF).

When this point is reached either the resistance or the way the exercise is done have to be modified in one way or another so that more repetitions can be done. That means that high-intensity training actually starts at a degree of

fatigue at which the set is usually terminated in conventional strength training (Robinson, 1990, p. 78).
In addition to the high-intensity bodybuilders purposely do not allow full recuperation between sets. They use incomplete breaks between sets as a way of realising an accumulation of fatigue. For many years high-volume, multiple-set training was the method of choice in bodybuilding and even today several authors still suggest a multiple-set approach for muscle building (Fleck & Kraemer, 1997; Stone et al., 1998; Zatsiorsky, 1995). It must be questioned whether it really is the high volume of bodybuilding training that is primarily responsible for the outstanding degree of muscular hypertrophy that can be realised by such training or if it is not rather the high training intensity that triggers muscle growth. Authors who try to prove the superiority of high-volume training for muscular growth by stating that this kind of volume is responsible for the enormous muscle mass achieved by bodybuilders often fail to mention that low-volume single-set training has been used very successfully by various bodybuilders.

Heavy Duty

Single-set training has been used in bodybuilding for many years. In 1980 Mentzer published his famous book "Heavy Duty" in which he advised bodybuilders to use single-set training for maximum muscle growth. Mentzer did not only suggest that one set per exercise should be performed, he went even further by suggesting that bodybuilders do only one set per muscle group taking each set to absolute failure incorporating several HITMs (table 2).

Table 2: Heavy-Duty-split recommended by Mentzer (1980)

first day	third day	fifth day
chest, shoulders and triceps	legs	back and biceps
pre-exhaustion exercise: flies followed by incline presses	pre-exhaustion exercise: leg extensions, barbell squat	pre-exhaustion exercise: pullovers, chin-ups
pre-exhaustion exercise: lateral dumbbell raises barbell press	pre-exhaustion exercise: leg curls, stiff-legged deadlift	pre-exhaustion exercise: scott curls, barbell curls
pre-exhaustion exercise: dips, triceps extensions at the lat pulldown machine	standing calf raises	
For the pre-exhaustion exercises a resistance is chosen that allows 8-RM to 10-RM. Immediately after failure has been reached on the pre-exhaustion exercises, the basic exercises are done with a weight that allows only five or six repetitions, followed by two or three forced reps and one or two negative reps.		

The HITM he considered to be the most important one is pre-exhaustion (Darden, 1983). Mentzer further suggested that bodybuilders applying his heavy duty method train less often in order to allow for more time for recuperation. However, when heavy duty training was dealt with in scientific journals, it was often reduced to the high-intensity aspects neglecting other decisive components like training volume and training frequency. Thus, "heavy duty" became a synonym for the kind of high-intensity training generally applied by bodybuilders. Mentzer himself applied his theories to his own training and won the prestigious "Mr. Universe" title. Most bodybuilders, however, were sceptical about the heavy duty concept and multiple-set training remained the predominant method for many years. One reason for the scepticism that heavy duty aroused among bodybuilders was that Mentzer's concept was strongly influenced by the theories of Arthur Jones who not only supported single-set training but also sold a special kind of training equipment (Nautilus) that was designed for single-set training. Consequently, single-set training was considered by many to be a way of promoting a certain training method in order to sell expensive training equipment that is supposed to be used for that kind of training.

> " ... the 'one-set-to-failure'-theory was devised by Arthur Jones to sell his expensive Nautilus machines to gym owners who had to have a high turnover of members to make any money. [They] could not have someone using a $2000 pullover machine for 5 sets of 10 reps." (Bass, 1999)

Even in the scientific community those allegations were made:

> "In the 1970s the pseudo science and marketing claims about weight training equipment and the associated philosophies to sell that equipment started to influence the decisions of strength coaches hungry for information." (Kraemer, 1997, p. 132)

Another factor that contributed tremendously to the predominance of multiple-set training was that competitive bodybuilding was dominated by athletes who applied the multiple-set approach to their own training and believed that their outstanding muscle mass was a result of high-volume training. Not only did those athletes use multiple-set training in their own training, they also recommended the high volume approach to other trainees:

> "... I recommend at least 20 sets total for most body parts (...) and at least 15 to 16 sets for the biceps and the same for the triceps." (Schwarzenegger, 1984, p. 195)

Heavy Duty vs. volume training

The heavy duty concept was quite well-known among bodybuilders during the 1980s but it was not used by many until some bodybuilders used this training approach and did well in professional bodybuilding competitions. The popularity of single-set training increased tremendously among bodybuilders when Dorian Yates, a professional Bodybuilder from Great Britain, applied Mentzer's theories to his own training and dominated competitive bodybuilding during the early 1990s by winning five consecutive "Mr. Olympia" competitions. In his book "Blood and Guts" he described his training programme which consisted of split workouts concentrating on basic exercises done for only one or two sets each and using high-intensity training methods in every working set (Yates, 1993; Yates & Wolff, 1993). In addition to those HITMs already described by Bührle and Werner (1984) he also recommends "rest-pause training" and "triple drops". Rest-pause training is also known as "extended sets". After the point of momentary muscular failure has been reached, the athlete re-racks the weight, pauses for a few seconds and then continues the set. This rest-pause technique can be repeated several times and is still counted as only one set. "Triple drops" are "descending sets" (Gaspari, 1990) during which the weight is reduced three times. The competitive success of bodybuilders who use heavy duty training has resulted in a dichotomy of recommendations concerning the adequate training volume for muscular hypertrophy. There are the advocates of multiple-set training who believe that single-set training may be appropriate for beginners or recreational athletes but does not provide a sufficient training stimulus for competitive athletes whereas advocates of single-set training are convinced that the low training volume of single-set training enables athletes to take each set to absolute muscular failure and thus provide the kind of stimulus necessary for muscular hypertrophy.

When single-set training became popular among bodybuilders in the 1990s, Mentzer argued that the growing acceptance of high-intensity low-volume training supported what he had been recommending for many years and published an updated version of his heavy duty concept (Mentzer, 1997, 1998). Because of this development the heavy duty concept has become well established among bodybuilders and the training methodology in bodybuilding is divided into heavy duty training which has bodybuilders do only one very intense set of each exercise and "volume training" (Kraemer et al., 1995, p. 195) which requires multiple sets of each exercise. Proponents of both training methods claim that there are scientific studies which demonstrate that their kind of training is the superior one. The fact that single-set training is being used successfully by numerous bodybuilders shows that the training methodology in bodybuilding can no longer be used as an argument for the superiority of high-volume training for muscular hypertrophy. Carpinelli and Otto (1998) point out that multiple-set training was believed by many to be superior and therefore became the method of choice although its superiority had not yet been proven. They review 33 studies which fail to prove the superiority of either approach. Philipp (1999b) argues that the results of those studies do not provide a final answer but either show that single-set training may produce which are at least comparable to those from multiple-set training (Messier & Dill, 1985; Miller et al., 1994; Starkey et al., 1996; Vincent et al., 1998) or seem to support the conclusion that multiple-set training provides superior results (Jacobson, 1986; Kramer et al., 1997; Marx et al., 1998; Sanborn et al., 1998).

It is also questionable whether the results of those studies can be compared with each other at all since they applied different levels of intensity. Philipp (1999a) compared single-set training with multiple-set training but only the single-set training was done with high-intensity using several HITMs and produced remarkably better results than the high-volume approach. This implies that the key factor for inducing muscular hypertrophy is the intensity at which a set is done rather than the number of sets. If the set is taken to the point of muscular failure or even beyond, one set is sufficient to stimulate muscular hypertrophy.

Another aspect that has to be taken into consideration in this context is the influence of different training volumes on the athletes' hormonal state. Usually this aspect is considered to support the superiority of multiple-set training because it has been shown to stimulate the secretion of endogenous anabolic hormones (Gotshalk et al., 1997; Marx et al., 1998; Mulligan, Fleck, Gordon,

Koziris, & Triplett-McBride, 1996). Crist (1992) therefore recommends six to eight sets per exercise for bodybuilders because he considers this high-volume approach to be ideal for inducing the maximal secretion of endogenous growth hormone. However, this kind of training volume will lead to overtraining in many athletes, especially when HITMs are applied. Ostrowski et al. (1997, pp. 153-154) discovered "a shift in the testosterone/cortison (anabolic/catabolic) ratio in some individuals, suggesting the possibility of overtraining" when only four sets per exercise were done which is only half of the volume that Christ recommends.

One factor that has been overestimated so far is training experience. It has often been stated that single-set training may be appropriate for beginners or recreational athletes whereas experienced athletes should increase their training volume (Kraemer, 1996, p. 196; Kramer et al., 1997, p. 143). Neither Ostrowski et al. (1997) whose subjects had all been training for at least one year found any proof for this statement nor did Hass, Garzarella, De Hoyos and Pollock (1998) who had two groups of experienced athletes either increase their training volume or continue to do only one set after one year of single-set training.

Despite the fact that all these findings are being discussed in the scientific community and among trainees world-wide, there are some aspects that are often neglected: One study that has been cited innumerable times because it is supposed to demonstrate the superiority of multiple-set training is the study by Berger (1962) who had his subjects perform different numbers of sets and reps of the bench press in order to find out which kind of training resulted in the greatest strength increase. He found the best improvements when three sets of six reps were done. Many times this study was misinterpreted as demonstrating that there is a proportional relationship between the number of sets and the strength increases. A close look at the results (table 3) shows that one set produced better results than two sets and that there is no proportional relationship between training volume and improvements in strength.

Table 3: Effect of varied weight training programs on strength (Berger, 1962)

sets	repetitions	strength increase (pounds)
3	6	161.3
1	6	156.1
2	10	155.8
3	2	153.8
3	10	153.1
2	6	152.9
1	10	151.3
1	2	149.2
2	2	145.8

The fact that "the practices of elite strength/power athletes" (Stone et al., 1998, p. 26) and bodybuilders in particular are still being used as an argument for the superiority of multiple-set training is quite questionable because many of those athletes are successfully using single-set training which makes undifferentiated statements pointless.

Finally, one aspect which is often overlooked is the total volume of a training session. Bodybuilders usually split their workouts and train one or two muscle groups per day. In each training session they do several exercises for the same muscle group in order to stimulate growth in as many parts of a muscle as possible (Antonio, 2000; Tanny, 1989). In contrary to that, Kramer et al. (1997) had their subjects only do one set per muscle group so that they did only a total of four sets in a workout training their legs, their shoulders, their chests, and their abdominal muscles.

Bodybuilders applying the single-set approach to their training, however, usually do one set of each exercise which does not necessarily mean that only one exercise per muscle group is done (Gießing, 2004).

Although the results of the current research cannot yet answer the question of which training volume is the ideal one for stimulating maximal muscular hypertrophy, they make one thing very obvious: If each working set is taken to the point of momentary muscular failure or beyond, single-set training may be just as effective as multiple-set training.

References

Antonio, J. (2000). Nonuniform response of skeletal muscle to heavy resistance training: Can bodybuilders induce regional muscle hypertrophy? *Journal of Strength and Conditioning Research, 14*(1), 102-113.

Bass, C. (1999). *New evidence on sets controversy,* 1999, from www.cbass.com/new´evides.html

Berger, R. A. (1962). Effect of varied weight training programs on strength. *The Research Quarterly, 33*(2), 168-181.

Bührle, M., & Werner, E. (1984). Das Muskelquerschnittstraining der Bodybuilder [Muscle-hypertrophy training by bodybuilders]. *Leistungssport, 14*(3), 5-9.

Carpinelli, R. N., & Otto, R. M. (1998). Strength training. Single versus multiple sets. *Sports Medicine, 26*(2), 73-84.

Crist, D. M. (1992). Gestaffeltes Volumentraining. Ein innovatives - und umstrittenes - Konzept für maximalen Muskelaufbau und minimales Risiko [Staggered volume training. An innovative - and controversial - concept for maximum muscle growth and minimum risk]. *Sportrevue, 11*, 96-98.

Darden, E. (1983). The pre-exhaustion principle in strength training. *Athletic Journal, 1*(46), 66-67.

Dudley, G. A., Tesch, P. A., Miller, B. J., & Buchanan, P. (1991). Importance of eccentric actions in performance adaptations to resistance training. *Aviation, Space & Environmental Medicine, 62*(6), 543-550.

Fleck, S. J., & Kraemer, W. J. (1987). *Designing resistance training programs* (1st ed.). Champaign, IL: Human Kinetics.

Fleck, S. J., & Kraemer, W. J. (1997). *Designing resistance training programs* (2nd ed.). Champaign, IL: Human Kinetics.

Gaspari, R. (1990). Descending sets. *Flex, 6*, 33.

Gießing, J. (2004). *1 Satz Training - Ein wissenschaftlich fundiertes Konzept für schnellstmöglichen Muskelaufbau im Bodybuilding [Single-set training. A concept for rapid muscle gains based on scientific findings]* (1st ed.). Arnsberg: Novagenics.

Gotshalk, L. A., Loebel, C. C., Nindl, B. C., Putukian, M., Sebastianelli, W. J., Newton, R. U., et al. (1997). Hormonal responses of multiset versus single-set heavy-resistance exercise protocols. *Canadian Journal of Applied Physiology, 22*(3), 244-255.

Hass, C. J., Garzarella, L., De Hoyos, D., & Pollock, M. L. (1998). Effects of training volume on strength and endurance in experienced resistance trained adults. *Medicine & Science in Sports & Exercise, 30*(5), 208-214.

Hemmling, G. (1994). *Anpassungen des neuromuskulären Systems an eine neuentwickelte Trainingsmethode [Adaptations of the neuromuscular systems to a newly developed training method].* Köln: Sport und Buch Strauß.

Jacobson, B. H. (1986). A comparison of two progressive weight training techniques on knee extensor strength. *Athletic Training, 21*(4), 315-318, 390.

Jones, D. A., & Rutherford, O. M. (1987). Human muscle strength training: the effects of three different regimens and the nature of the resultant changes. *Journal of Physiology, 391*, 1-11.

Koch, A., & Haff, G. G. (1999). Training for size vs. training for power. *Muscular Development, 33*(8), 96-103.

Kraemer, W. J. (1996). Myths and Resistance Training, Part I. *Muscular Development, 34*(2), 148-149, 194-196.

Kraemer, W. J. (1997). A series of studies - the physiological basis for strength training in American football: fact over philosophy. *Journal of Strength and Conditioning Research, 11*(3), 131-142.

Kraemer, W. J., Newton, N., Bush, M., Volek, V., Triplett, N., & Koziris, J. (1995). Varied multiple set resistance training programs produce greater gains than single set program. *Medicine & Science in Sports & Exercise, 7*(5), S195.

Kramer, J. B., Stone, M. H., O'Bryant, H. S., Conley, M. S., Johnson, R. L., Nieman, D. C., et al. (1997). Effects of single vs. multiple sets of weight training: impact of volume, intensity, and variation. *Journal of Strength and Conditioning Research, 11*(3), 143-147.

Marx, J. O., Nindl, B. C., Gotshalk, L. A., Volek, J. S., Harmann, F. S., Dohi, K., et al. (1998). The effects of a low-volume progressive resistance exercise program versus a high-volume periodized resistance exercise program on muscular perfomance in women. In K. Häkkinen & (Hrsg.) (Eds.), *International conference on weightlifting and strength training* (pp. 167-168). Lathi, Finland: Gummerus Printing.

Mentzer, M. (1980). *Heavy duty*. Venice.

Mentzer, M. (1991). Realistic expectations. *Flex, 2*, 67-69.

Mentzer, M. (1997). *Heavy duty II. Mind and body*. Venice.

Mentzer, M. (1998). Mike Mentzer´s new advanced high intensity training program. *Muscular Development, 35*(5), 134-139.

Messier, S. P., & Dill, M. E. (1985). Alterations in strength and maximal oxygen uptake consequent to Nautilus circuit weight training. *Research Quarterly for Exercise and Sport, 56*(4), 345-351.

Miller, J. P., Pratley, R. E., Goldberg, A. P., Gordon, P., Rubin, M., Treuth, M. S., et al. (1994). Strength training increases insulin action in healthy 50- to 65-yr-old men. *Journal of Applied Physiology, 77*(3), 1122-1127.

Mulligan, S., Fleck, S., Gordon, S., Koziris, L., & Triplett-McBride, N. (1996). Influence of resistance exercise volume on growth hormone and cortisol concentrations in women. *Journal of Strength and Conditioning Research, 10*(4), 256-262.

Ostrowski, K. J., Wilson, G. J., Weatherby, R., Murphy, P. W., & Lyttle, A. D. (1997). The effect of weight training volume on hormonal output and muscular size and function. *Journal of Strength and Conditioning Research, 11*(3), 148-154.

Philipp, M. (1999a). Ein Satz genügt! - Erfahrungen mit Mehrsatz- und Einsatz-Methoden im Krafttraining. Eine Fallstudie als Diskussionsbeitrag zur Anregung von Werner Kieser [One set is enough! - Experiences with multilpe-set and single-set training in strength training. A case study to adress the controversy with Werner Kieser]. *Leistungssport, 29*(1), 26-28.

Philipp, M. (1999b). Einsatz-Training versus Mehrsatz-Training. Zur Kontroverse um die Satzzahl beim Krafttraining unter Berücksichtigung empirischer Evidenzen [Single-set versus multiple-set training. To adress the controversy under consideration of empirical data]. *Leistungssport, 29*(4), 27-34.

Robinson, E. (1990). Training past failure. *Flex, 8*, 76-78.

Sanborn, K., Boros, R., Hruby, J., Schilling, B., O´Bryant, H., Johnson, R., et al. (1998). Performance effecte of weigth training with multiple sets not to failure versus a single set to failure in women: a prelimenary study. In K. Häkkinen (Ed.), *International conference on weigthlifting and strength training* (pp. 157-158). Lathi, Finnland: Gummerus Printing.

Schwarzenegger, A. (1984). *Arnold´s bodybuilding for men*. New York.

Starkey, D. B., Pollock, M. L., Ishida, Y., Welsch, M. A., Brechue, W. F., Graves, J. E., et al. (1996). Effect of resistance training volume on strength and muscle thickness. *Medicine & Science in Sports & Exercise, 28*(10), 1311-1320.

Stone, M. H., Plisk, S. S., Stone, M. E., Schilling, B. K., O´Bryant, H. S., & Pierce, K. C. (1998). Athletic performance development: Volume load-1 set vs. multiple sets, training velocity and training variation. *Strength and Conditioning Journal, 20*(6), 22-31.

Tanny, A. (1989). Target training. *Muscle & Fitness, 2*, 126-128.

Vincent, K., De Hoyos, D., Garzarella, L., Hass, C., Nordman, M., & Pollock, M. L. (1998). Relationship between indices of knee extension strength before and after training. *Medicine & Sciene in Sports & Exercise, 30*(5), S163.

Yates, D. (1993). The one set per movement routine. *Flex, 1*, 72-75, 112-114.

Yates, D., & Wolff, B. (1993). *Blood and Guts. The ultimate approach to building maximum muscle mass*. Woodland Hills.

Zatsiorsky, V. M. (1995). *Science and practice of strength training*. Champaign, IL: Human Kinetics.

WOLFGANG KEMMLER, DIRK LAUBER, SIMON VON STENGEL &
KLAUS ENGELKE

Developing maximum strength in older adults - a series of studies

Keywords: periodized training, single-set training, perceived exertion, training volume, multiple-set training

Introduction

The reduction of muscle mass is a major component of normal aging (ACSM, 1998a). Between 50 and 70 years of age a loss of ≈30 % in maximum strength can be observed (ACSM, 1998a). The consequences associated with the ongoing decline of strength are complex and far reaching. With respect to fractures that are a central risk factor of the elderly, maximum strength is associated with both, falls (Kenny, Rubenstein, Martin, & Tinetti, 2001) and bone mineral density (Burr, 1997). Thus, resistance training has been recommended by major health organisations for improving health and fitness (ACSM, 1998a, 1998b; Kohrt, Bloomfield, Little, Nelson, & Yingling, 2004).
However, training concepts for healthy elderly persons differ widely from those for athletes. The training volume of ambulatory courses is restricted to a maximum of 2 - 3 sessions per week due to the reluctance of most subjects to spend a large amount of their free time for prevention (Marcus, 1998). In order to achieve an optimum effect despite the limited possibility of manipulating all training variables, modern training strategies have to be used to ensure a stable effect on strength development. So far controversy still exists which exercise program most favourably affects maximum strength in older non-athletic subjects (ACSM, 1998b). The current study was conducted to separately determine the effect of the following three different resistance exercise strategies on maximum strength (1-RM) in trained postmenopausal women:

1. Non-linear versus linear periodized training,
2. single versus multiple-set resistance training,
3. load prescription versus perceived exertion protocols.

For each trial a cross-over design in which each subject served as its own control was chosen.

Material and Methods

Subjects

76 subjects of the training arm of the Erlangen Fitness Osteoporosis Prevention Study (EFOPS) participated in the study. All subjects were early-postmenopausal (1 - 8 years postmenopausal), osteopenic and free of medication affecting bone or muscle metabolism (i.e. glucocorticoids, HRT). For a detailed description of recruiting and selection modalities the reader is kindly referred to our previous publications (Kemmler et al., 2002; Kemmler, Engelke et al., 2004; Kemmler, Lauber, von Stengel et al., 2005).

The EFOPS-study was approved by the ethics committee of the University of Erlangen (Ethik Antrag 905), the Bundesamt für Strahlenschutz (S9108-202/97/1, S21-22112-81-00) and the Bayerische Landesamt für Arbeitssicherheit (13B/3443-4/5/98). All study participants gave written informed consent.

Training program

The EFOPS program is a general purpose exercise program for older adults with emphasis on strength training. The exercise program consisted of two supervised group sessions and two home training sessions. The strength training sequence was spread out over the two joint training sessions: Session 1 was performed on machines (Technogym, Gambettola, Italy), the session 2 consisted of dumbbell and weighted vests exercises. The following dynamic exercises were performed during the high-intensity training periods: horizontal leg press, leg curls, bench press, rowing, leg adduction and abduction, abdominal flexion, back extension, lat pulley, leg extension, shoulder raises (all on resistance machines), squats/deadlifts, wide grip bench press, and 1 arm dumbbell rowing. Movements were performed in a 2-second (concentric), 1-second (static), 2-second (eccentric) mode with 90 - 120 s rest periods between the sets.

During the first 7 - 8 months of the EFOPS-study exercise intensity of the training was increased slowly up to 70 % 1-RM. During this preparatory phase the exercise intensity of the resistance training was controlled and adjusted every 6 to 8 weeks using 1-RM tests.

Month 8 - 9 of the study was used to introduce the periodized individual training logs. Calculation of training loads and repetitions from 1-RM values (instead of calculating 1-RM from repetitions to fatigue, RTF) were conducted using the equation of O´Conner, Simmons and O´Shea (1989) that was tested to be most adequate for our cohort (Kemmler, Lauber, Mayhew, & Wassermann, 2005).

Testing and procedures

As mentioned above, the first of the three trails reported here began 8 - 9 months after the start of the EFOPS study. Thus all participants were already trained. Study participants exercised in six different training groups. For the purpose of all three trials the training groups were randomly assigned to two groups. Besides the cross-over design and the stringent exclusion criteria's of the EFOPS study (Kemmler et al., 2002; Kemmler, Engelke et al., 2004; Kemmler, Lauber, von Stengel et al., 2005) both exercise subgroups (EG1 and EG2) were well-matched with respect to age, anthropometric variables, menopausal status, and nutritional intake (table 1).

Table 1: Baseline data for anthropometric and nutritional intake parameters

parameter	EG 1 (n = 39)	EG 2 (n = 37)	p
age [y]	55.8 ± 3.2	56.0 ± 3.2	n.s.
height [cm]	163.6 ± 6.7	164.1 ± 6.8	n.s.
weight [kg]	66.9 ± 8.8	68.0 ± 8.9	n.s.
body fat [%]	35.8 ± 5.1	36.3 ± 4.9	n.s.
LBM [kg]	42.1 ± 3.5	43.1 ± 2.9	n.s.
energy intake [kJ/d]	7767 ± 1283	7702 ± 1317	n.s.
vitamin D intake [µg/d]	5.3 ± 5.0	4.7 ± 5.2	n.s.

Table 2 shows the study profile. The three trials were separated by 5 weeks of non-periodized low-intensity resistance exercise and 1 - 2 weeks of rest.

Table 2: Study profile; TP: transition phase; LI: low-intensity resistance training; R=rest; mo: months, w: weeks; T: 1-RM-tests

trial 1			TP	trial 2			TP	trial 3		
period 1	LI	period 2	LI+R	period 1	LI	period 2	LI+R	period 1	LI	period 2
3 mo	5 w	3 mo	7 w	3 mo	5 w	3 mo	7 w	3 mo	5 w	3 mo
T	T T		T T		T T		T T		T T	T

As an example table 3 shows the profile of trial one. 5 weeks of non-periodized low-intensity training were performed between the high-intensity periods. Figure 1 illustrates results of the cross-over design using again trail one outcome variables.

Table 3: Example profile of trial one (LI: low-intensity resistance training)

time course	period 1 (weeks 1 - 12)	LI (weeks 13 - 17)	period 2 (weeks 18 - 29)
group 1 (EG 1)	periodized high-intensity regime 1	non-periodized low-intensity training	periodized high-intensity regime 2
group 2 (EG 2)	periodized high-intensity regime 2		periodized high-intensity regime 1

For all three trails compliance and attendance were assessed using individual training logs and attendance lists. Subjects that failed to participate in at least 20 out of 24 possible training sessions in any of the two periods were excluded from the analysis.

1-RM tests of horizontal leg press, seated bench press, rowing, and leg adduction were performed according to the protocol suggested by Kraemer et al. (1991). Proper conduct and maximum effort during the tests were controlled by research assistants. The reproducibility of our 1-RM protocol was tested after 6, 26 and 36 months of the EFOPS-study. Coefficient of variation (CV) was < 6 % for all test exercises for the first measurement and < 4 % for the second and third test. The tests were always performed in the last and first sessions of the low-intensity training periods bracketing the high-intensity periods (table 2).

Statistical analysis

For all three trials identical analysis procedures were used. Statistics were calculated using SPSS 12.0 (SPSS Inc., Chicago IL, USA). All measured values are reported as mean values (MV) and standard deviations (SD).

For normally distributed variables differences within and between groups were assessed with paired t-tests. Otherwise the Wilcoxon-test or Mann-Whitney U-test was used. Additionally between-group differences were analyzed using an analysis of variance (ANOVA) with repeated measurement design. All tests were t-tailed, a 5 %-probability-level was considered significant (*).

To determine the effect of the two competing protocols in each of the three trials (linear vs. non-linear; single-set vs. multiple-set; load prescription vs. perceived exertion), we calculated average changes in both groups by averaging the results from high-intensity periods 1 and 2. Thus, using the example of the single-set versus multiple-set trial (figure 1), the change of the single-set training is the average of the change of Group 2 during period 1 and of the change of Group 1 during period 2. Equivalently the change of the multiple-set protocol is average of the change of group 1 during period 1 and of the change of group 2 during period 2.

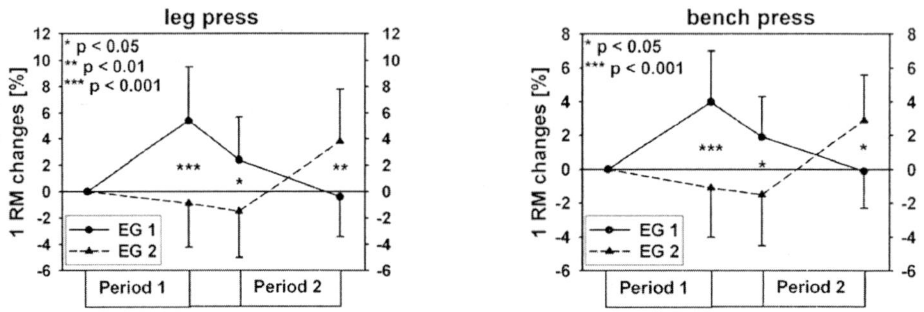

Figure 1: 1-RM development of leg and bench press for groups 1 and 2 during the 29 weeks of trial 1. EG 1 started with the multiple-set, EG 2 with the single-set protocol. Changes were also determined for 1-RM rowing and leg adduction (Kemmler, Lauber, Engelke, & Weineck, 2004). Significance of changes not shown in graphs

Trial 1: Effect of linear versus non-linear periodization

Introduction

After 7 - 8 months of exercise we observed a leveling-off effect of the 1-RM development in two out of four test exercises (non-significant differences compared with the previous test). Although there is still controversy whether periodization is superior to traditional (non-periodized) resistance training to increase 1-RM (review in ACSM, 2002; Carpinelli, Otto, & Winett, 2004; Fleck, 1999; Haff, 2004a, 2004b; Stone et al., 2000), at this point in time we decided to introduce periodized high-intensity protocols to provoke further adaptations. It was not an aim of this trial to evaluate the effect of meso-/microcycle periodization versus traditional resistance training programs on 1-RM. We rather wanted to compare two concepts of periodization, linear and non-linear (undulating).

Linear periodization is characterized by high initial volume and low-intensity. Volume decreases and intensity increases as training progresses. Each training phase is designed to focus on a particular physiological adaptation (ACSM, 2002). Non-linear or undulating periodization varies the volume and intensity of training more frequently. Heavy, moderate and light intensities of training can be alternated during each week of the month. Non-linear periodization models are preferred in sports with frequent competitions (Hoffman, 2002).

One may argue that the comparison of linear and non-linear periodization in non-athletic, postmenopausal women is rather sophisticated; however, we conducted this trial for the following reasons:

(1) Given the fact that generally only a limited number of training variables can be manipulated in preventional strength training for older subjects, it is important to identify general strategies that increase the effectiveness of the training. Further, given the necessity of a steady development of strength over many years, the collection and application of diverse effective training models is rational.
(2) Besides strength, endurance, balance and reaction are also relevant for the older adult. Thus it is important to determine whether non-linear protocols that allow to regularly increase the intensity of other training sequences focusing on these other skills are equally effective to increase 1-RM compared to linear periodization protocols.

Trial specific materials and methods

Trial 1 started 8 - 9 months after the start of the EFOPS-study. 76 subjects of the training arm of the EFOPS-study participated. Three participants dropped out during the trial. 20 subjects were excluded from the analysis due to poor attendance (< 20 out of 24 sessions). No differences between baseline data (table 1) of anthropometric and nutritional intake parameters and the corresponding data of trial 1 were observed. Table 4 shows 1-RM baseline values.

Table 4: Baseline 1-RM values for trial 1

parameter	EG 1 (n = 28)	EG 2 (n = 25)	p
leg press [kg]	153.5 ± 20.9	166.7 ± 20.3	n.s.
bench press [kg]	42.7 ± 5.2	44.0 ± 5.5	n.s.
rowing [kg]	42.8 ± 5.1	43.7 ± 5.1	n.s.
leg adduction [kg]	40.3 ± 6.8	42.6 ± 7.1	n.s.

In the linear periodized protocol (LP) intensity was linearly increased every week over a period of 6 weeks, with two peaks during the 12-week period (figure 2). In the non-linear periodization protocol (NLP) intensity and volume varied frequently. In addition the non-linear periodization included daily undulating periodization (5 % of the 1-RM, not recognizable in figure 2) within the microcycle, (i.e. Monday: 67.5 % 1-RM, Thursday: 72.5 % 1-RM). In the LP intensity and volume were stable during the microcycle (i.e. 70 % 1-RM for both sessions).
Figure 2 shows the training protocols for the session on resistance machines. Protocols for dumbbell and weighted vests exercises were designed equivalently. During this trial we did not maximize the number of repetitions to achieve complete exhaustion of the participants. In order to be able to associ-

ate the measured effect exclusively with the periodization and not to higher intensity or volume, training volume (repetitions/period) and relative intensity (average % 1-RM/period) were comparably designed for both groups (with slightly higher volume for the NLP). At baseline, group 1 started with the NLP, group 2 exercised with the LP. After 12 weeks of training and a low-intensity regenerational period of 5 weeks the cross-over design was realized. Group 1 performed the LP, group 2 crossed over to the NLP.

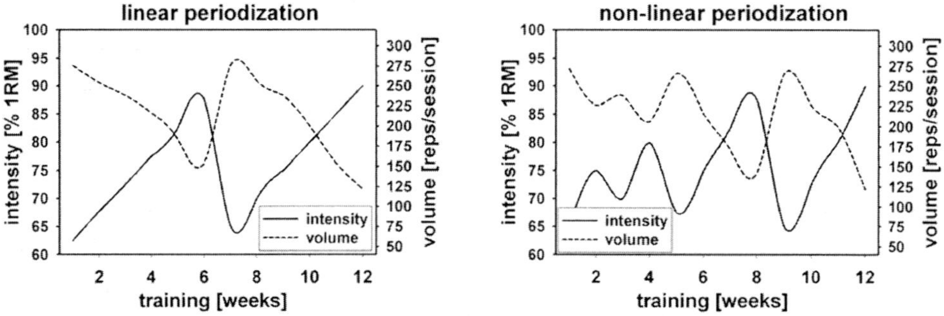

Figure 2: Intensity (% 1-RM) and volume (repetitions/session) on resistance machines. Equivalent protocols were used for weighted vest/dumbbell exercises

Results

1-RM changes averaged for both groups as described in the statistical analysis section are shown in figure 3. The changes of all test exercises were significant for both protocols. Between the protocols no significant differences were determined.

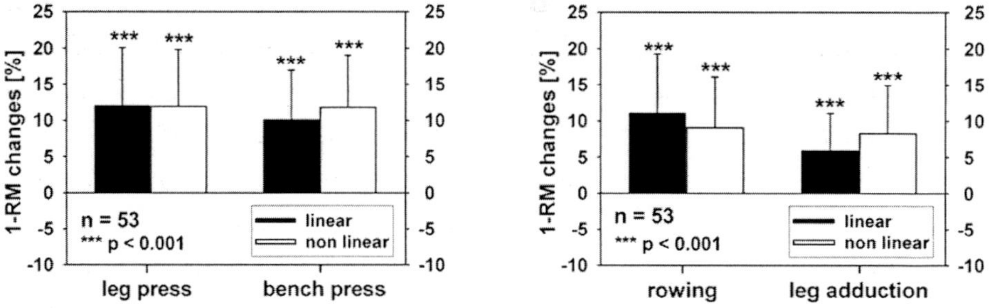

Figure 3: Average 1-RM changes for linear versus non-linear periodization

Trial specific discussion

A goal of periodization is to optimize training during short (weeks/months) as well as during long periods (years, olympic cycles, entire career) (Fleck, 1999). In this trial we focused on short term (12 weeks) periodization effects on 1-RM. Further, although a large variety of training variables can be manipulated, comparable to most other studies, the present study focused on the variation of intensity and volume. Two different regimes were compared, a linear periodized (LP) versus a non-linear periodized protocol (NLP).

However, our LP differs from the LP-protocols applied by other authors (i.e. Baker, Wilson, & Carlyon, 1994; Rhea, Ball, Phillips, & Burkett, 2002; Rhea, Landers, Alvar, & Arent, 2003; Stone et al., 2000). Rather than making changes over a period of months we manipulated intensity and volume on a weekly base. Further, contrarily to other linear protocols the structure of our protocol was undulatory. Thus our LP possesses some attributes of non-linear periodization. However, after the stepwise intensity increment (every 6 - 8 weeks) during the first 8 - 9 months of the EFOPS-study we decided to manipulate intensity and volume at least weekly to differ from the initial training protocol.

Comparing the design of both protocols, intensity and volume differed from session to session in the NLP, but on a weekly base in the LP. Further, variations of intensity/volume of the NLP were created more undulating compared with the LP. However, both protocols did not relevantly differ for total volume and total intensity.

With respect to 1-RM changes differences between the NLP and LP protocols we not observed. It is difficult to compare our result with other studies (Baker et al., 1994; Rhea, Ball et al., 2002; Stone et al., 2000) because of the different protocols applied. Two studies (Baker et al., 1994; Stone et al., 2000) confirmed our finding that LP and NLP were equally effective to increase 1-RM in trained subjects. However, in one of these studies (Stone et al., 2000) training volume significantly differed between LP and NLP with lower volume in NLP. In young male subjects with a minimum of two years of weight-training experience Rhea, Ball et al., (2002) compared the effect of LP (stepwise increment of intensity every 4 weeks) vs. daily undulating periodized programs on 1-RM and demonstrated significant differences for leg press (LP: +14 % vs. NLP: +29 %) and bench press (LP: +26 % vs. NLP: +56 % (!)).

It is difficult to explain the discrepancy between their and our results but our LP with weekly undulating periodization may be more effective than the LP of Rhea, Ball et al., (2002) although their 1-RM-changes were far higher ours. Thus, although our results demonstrate that our LP and NLP were equally effective to increase maximum strength in elderly subject, we cannot generalize this conclusion for other protocols or cohorts.

Trial 2: Effect of single versus multiple-sets of exercise

Introduction

The background of this trial was rather pragmatic. Taken into account that early-postmenopausal women with a variety of risk factors but without severe complaints are unwilling to spend a large amount of time for preventional activities, the available time should be utilized most effectively. Single-set training regimens save time (Messier & Dill, 1985) that could be spent for other relevant training contents. However, although a large number of studies focus on the single-set vs. multiple-set issue (review in Carpinelli & Otto, 1998; Feigenbaum & Pollock, 1997; Galvao & Taaffe, 2004; Rhea, Alvar, Burkett, & Ball, 2003; Wolfe, LeMura, & Cole, 2004), there is no unequivocal vote. Unfortunately this discrepancy is difficult to resolve because a large variety of causes may contribute. Exercise studies comparing single- and multiple-set protocols not only differ with respect to training volume but also in regard to investigated muscle groups (Nicklas et al., 1995; Ryan, Pratley, Elahi, & Goldberg, 1995), exercise mode, i.e. velocity (Marx et al., 2001; Sanborn et al., 2000; Stone, Johnson, & Carter, 1979), exercise intensity (Capen, 1956; Marx et al., 2001; Messier & Dill, 1985), work until failure or not (Kramer et al., 1997), periodization strategy (Kraemer et al., 2000; Marx et al., 2001), and equipment used for the measurements (i.e. Messier & Dill, 1985; Stone et al., 1979). Further, with one exception (Ryan et al., 1995), all studies included young or middle-aged subjects.

All these factors may affect maximum strength changes induced by the exercise protocol and must be carefully accounted for in the study design or data analysis (Rhea, Alvar, Ball, & Burkett, 2002). Thus, in this trial we focused on comparable conditions in both subgroups (single-set vs. multiple-set) to clarify the issue which training strategy is more effective to increase 1-RM in trained older subjects.

Trial specific materials and methods

Trial 2 started 18 months after the start of the EFOPS-study. 71 subjects of the training arm of the EFOPS-study participated. None of the participants dropped out. 21 subjects were excluded from the analysis due to poor attendance. No differences between baseline data (table 1) of anthropometric and nutritional intake parameters and the corresponding data of trial 2 were observed. Further, with the exception of the baseline 1-RM leg press values (table 5) confounding factors were comparable for both groups. For more specific details of the trial the reader is kindly referred to another publication (Kemmler, Lauber et al., 2004). Table 5 shows 1-RM baseline values.

Table 5: Baseline 1-RM values for trial 2

parameter	EG 1 (n = 29)	EG 2 (n = 21)	p
leg press [kg]	163.1 ± 22.1	182.6 ± 19.7	*
bench press [kg]	45.2 ± 5.7	47.0 ± 5.7	n.s.
rowing [kg]	45.0 ± 5.1	45.5 ± 5.1	n.s.
leg adduction [kg]	41.3 ± 7.9	44.8 ± 7.9	n.s.

Single-set training was defined as one set per exercise per session, multiple-set training included 2 - 4 set per exercise per session (figure 4). Apart from this difference all training and test parameters were identical between groups. During this trial we did not maximize the number of repetitions to achieve complete exhaustion of the participants.

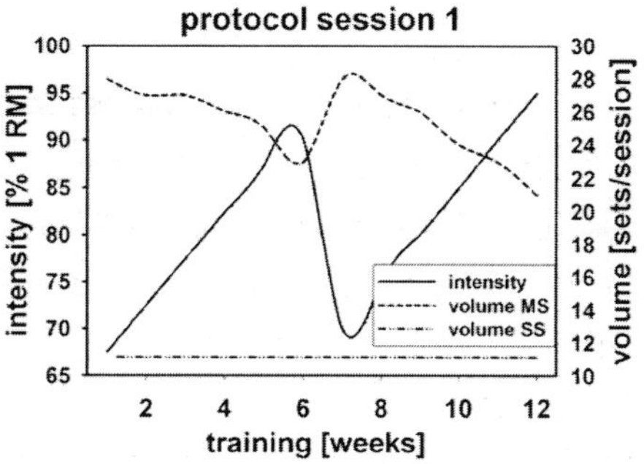

Figure 4: Intensity as percentage of the 1-RM and volume in sets / session of the strength training part on resistance machines. Equivalent protocols were used for weighted vest/dumbbell exercises

At baseline, group 1 started with the multiple-set protocol, group 2 exercised with the single-set protocol. After 12 weeks of training and a low-intensity regenerational period of 5 weeks the cross-over design was realized. Group 1 performed the single-set regime group 2 crossed over to the multiple-set program.

Results

1-RM changes averaged for both groups as described in statistical analysis section are shown in figure 5. Changes of 1-RM for all exercises were significantly higher for the multiple-set protocol compared with the single-set protocol.

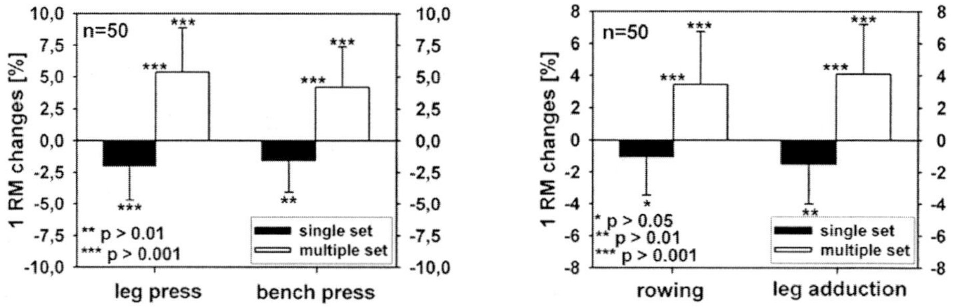

Figure 5: Average 1-RM changes for multiple-set and single-set training

Trial specific discussion

Our results clearly indicate that a multiple-set regime is superior to a single-set regime to increase 1-RM in trained postmenopausal women. Generally our results are in accordance with the literature. Differences between single- and multiple-set protocols are far more obvious in trained subjects or athletes than in untrained subjects (Kraemer, 1997; Kraemer et al., 2000; Kramer et al., 1997; Rhea, Alvar et al., 2002; Schlumberger, Stec, & Schmidtbleicher, 2001; Wolfe et al., 2004). Our trial 2 extends these results to trained older (female) subjects.

Trial 3: Effect of load prescription vs. perceived exertion protocols

Introduction

The mode of prescribing exercise intensity is a central determinant of resistance programs. Generally two strategies exist: (1) prescription of load as a percentage of the 1-RM. This mode is typically used to increase athletic performance (LeSuer, McCormick, Mayhew, Wasserstein, & Arnold, 1997; Mayhew, Clemens et al., 1995). (2) perceived exertion rates as utilized in resistance exercise for health and fitness (Buskies & Boeckh-Behrens, 1999; Gearhart et al., 2002; Pincivero, Coelho, & Campy, 2003). From a scientific point of view the first alternative should be favored (Ehlenz, Grosser, & Zimmermann, 1998; Weineck, 2000) but limitations may prevent the application of 1-RM based load prescription protocols in the health and fitness domain. Besides risk of injuries, compliance, equipment, and assignment of the 1-RM-values (Fröhlich, Schmidtbleicher, & Emrich, 2002; Gießing, 2003) the major limitation to prescribe loads is the increased expenditure induced by 1-RM tests and calculations. Obviously the protocol decision should primarily be based on the effect of the protocol rather than on expenditure. Thus, the purpose of this trial was to determine the effect of a load prescription protocol versus a perceived exertion protocol on 1-RM in trained postmenopausal women.

Trial specific materials and methods

Trial 3 started 27 months after the start of the EFOPS-study. 67 subjects of the training arm of the EFOPS-study participated. None of the participants dropped out, but only 49 subjects fulfilled training attendance criterion in both, the load prescription and the perceived exertion protocol. No differences between baseline data (table 1) of anthropometric and nutritional intake parameters and the corresponding data of trial 3 were observed. Further, confounding factors were comparable for both groups both. More specific details of this trial were published elsewhere (Kemmler, Lauber, Weineck et al., 2005). Table 6 shows 1-RM baseline values.

Table 6: Baseline 1-RM values for trial 3

parameter	EG 1 (n = 26)	EG 2 (n = 23)	p
leg press [kg]	172.7 ± 20.7	179.6 ± 19.9	n.s.
bench press [kg]	46.1 ± 5.5	47.3 ± 5.2	n.s.
rowing [kg]	45.9 ± 5.0	46.4 ± 5.1	n.s.
leg adduction [kg]	43.3 ± 7.4	44.8 ± 7.3	n.s.

Both protocols were identically structured and periodized according to the multiple-set protocol described in figure 3 with the exception of the loads that were given in the load prescription protocol and that should have been adequately selected in the perceived exertion protocol. Thus both protocols focused on work to complete fatigue ("forced last repetition"). The load prescription protocol was based on the equation of O`Conner et al. (1989), which was tested to be the most adequate equation for our cohort (Kemmler, Lauber, Mayhew et al., 2005). Subjects performing the perceived exertion protocol were told to select a load that allowed the given number of repetitions when working to fatigue.

Group 1 started with the load prescription protocol, group 2 performed the perceived exertion regime during the first 12 weeks of the trial. After 4 weeks of low-intensity regenerational training the cross-over design was realized. Group 1 performed the perceived exertion protocol, group 2 crossed over to the load prescription protocol.

Results

1-RM changes averaged for both groups as described in statistical analysis section are shown in figure 6. Although 1-RM-changes for all exercises were higher for the load prescription protocol, significant changes could be observed for bench press only.

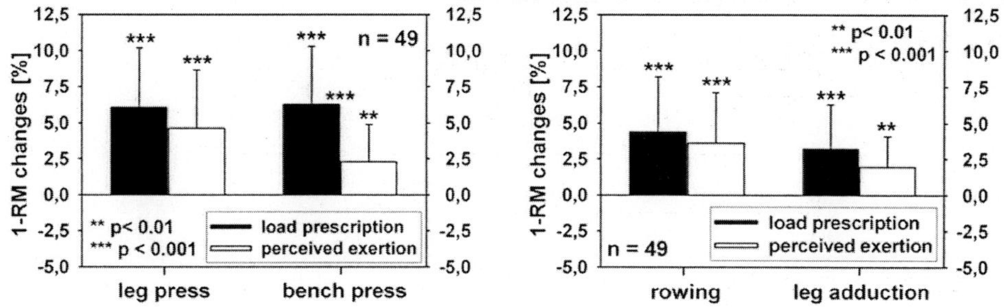

Figure 6: Average 1-RM changes for load prescription versus perceived exertion

Trial specific discussion

Again the purpose of the present trial was rather pragmatic. Under the premise that load prescription protocols are more elaborate than perceived exertion protocols, the effectiveness of load prescription protocols on 1-RM should be superior to perceived exertion protocols. However, our trial did not show a general superiority of load prescription protocols. Both protocols significantly increased 1-RM of all test exercises with significant protocol differences for bench press only. Thus, both programs were adequate to increase 1-RM in trained postmenopausal women.

Contrarily, Glass and Stanton (2004) reported that self-selected training intensity was not adequate to induce subsequent strength increases. Although subjects were told to "choose a load that you feel will be sufficient to improve your muscular strength" male and female participants of the study selected training loads that were not sufficient to induce strength gains. However, there are two main differences between Glass and Stanton's and our study. Firstly, their cohort were novice weightlifters with no previous weightlifting experience, while our subjects that were trained with load prescription protocol before, were able to select an adequate load for a given number of repetitions. Also our "work to fatigue strategy" was easier to realize than the more abstract aforementioned instruction given by Glass and Stanton (2004).

Thus despite our results, we recommend to regularly implement load prescription protocols to increase the participant's awareness of their individual load/repetition relationship. This recommendation is in particular valid for resistance training novices.

General comments

In this article three aspects of resistance training strategies were addressed. The trails were embedded in the overall EFOPS training design. Therefore starting with limitations of the investigation reported here, it must be mentioned that EFOPS did not focus exclusively on resistance training. 20 - 25 min of aerobics and multidirectional jumps were performed before the resistance sequence. Also the low-intensity training periods were not long enough to induce a wash-out of the strength gains of the previous high-intensity period. Thus, sequence effects may have affected our results. Another limitation may be the use of average 1-RM changes as primary endpoint because as outlined in the Statistcs section these changes were averaged over two periods. Although we are aware that this may not be the optimum solution, we abstained from more sophisticated analysis.
Our study also possesses several strengths: (1) Our cohort was a homogeneous group of pre-trained early postmenopausal women. (2) Confounding effects like nutrition, anthropometric- and life style changes, medication and diseases were strictly controlled. Subjects with relevant changes during the study course (Kemmler, Engelke et al., 2004; Kemmler, Lauber, von Stengel et al., 2005) were excluded from the analysis (3) Groups were randomly assigned to the protocols and due to the cross-over design subjects served as their own control. Thus, group differences should not have biased our results. (4) Subjects with low compliance and attendance were excluded from the analysis. (5) The number of approximately 50 included subjects was high enough to detect relevant differences between protocols.
All protocols with the exception of the perceived exertion protocol were based on the calculation of training loads from 1-RM values using the equation of O´Conner et al. (1989). It has been pointed out that in general the conduction of regular 1-RM tests in non-athletic resistance training may be difficult due to the following reasons: (1) An increased potential for injuries by the use of heavy loads (Mayhew, Ball, Busby, Arnold, & Bowen, 1992; Mayhew, Prinster et al., 1995). (2) Problems due to test compliance. (3) The time effort for the preparation of a 1-RM test. (4) The disruption of training continuity. Further, although numerous equations were developed and tested with different cohorts (Wood, Maddalozzo, & Harter, 2002), no equation exists that focuses on trained older women. Finally, some authors indicated that the association be-

tween 1-RM and corresponding repetitions to fatique (RTF) varied among different resistance exercises (Buskies & Boeckh-Behrens, 1999; Hoeger, Baratte, Hale, & Hopkins, 1987, 1990; Marschall & Fröhlich, 1999).

Although we do not want to negate all the above mentioned limitations we do not agree with the more critical concerns regarding 1-RM-tests or the transformation of 1-RM values into RTF ranges.

Although we performed a plethora of 1-RM tests during the last 3 years we did not observe any injury which was related to the use of maximum loads. Also, regarding the transformation of 1-RM to RTF values, present equations can be tested for the own cohort when additionally performing RTF-tests. For our cohort the equation of O´Conner et al. (1989) was adequate with a mean value of the absolute value of the difference between 1-RM and predicted 1-RM of < 4 % for all test exercises (Kemmler, Lauber, Mayhew et al., 2005). Further, we did not detect relevant differences in the association between 1-RM and corresponding RTF among our test exercises.

In summary our results confirm that in trained postmenopausal women:

1. Single-set periodized strength training regimes are less effective in producing 1-RM improvements than periodized multiple-set strength training regimes.
2. Both linear and non-linear strength training periodization patterns can be used successfully to produce significant 1-RM strength improvements with no significant differences between both patterns.
3. RPE based periodized strength training strategies enabling participants to self-select training loads can be successfully used to produce significant 1-RM gains, with no significant differences in comparison to more time consuming load prescription-based periodized strength training strategies.

Our trials indicate that performance-orientated strength training strategies, mainly derived from competitive sports, can very well be induced in nowadays preventive strength training work with elderly women. This adds variety and effectiveness to ambulatory training programmes that are usually limited in training volume.

References

ACSM. (1998a). Exercise and physical activity for older adults. *Medicine & Science in Sports & Exercise, 30*(6), 992-1008.

ACSM. (1998b). The recommended quantity and quality of exercise for developing and maintaining cardiorespiratory and muscular fitness, and flexibility in healthy adults. *Medicine & Science in Sports & Exercise, 30*(6), 975-991.

ACSM. (2002). Progression models in resistance training for healthy adults. *Medicine & Science in Sports & Exercise, 34*(2), 364-380.

Baker, D., Wilson, G., & Carlyon, R. (1994). Periodization: The effect on strength of manipulating volume and intensity. *Journal of Strength and Conditioning Research, 8*(4), 235-242.

Burr, D. B. (1997). Muscle strength, bone mass, and age-related bone loss. *Journal of Bone and Mineral Research, 12*(10), 1547-1551.

Buskies, W., & Boeckh-Behrens, W.-U. (1999). Probleme bei der Steuerung der Trainingsintensität im Krafttraining auf der Basis von Maximalkrafttests [Problems concerning the management of training intensity in strength training]. *Leistungssport, 29*(3), 4-8.

Capen, E. K. (1956). Study of four programs of heavy resistance exercises for development of muscular strength. *The Research Quarterly, 27*(2), 132-142.

Carpinelli, R. N., & Otto, R. M. (1998). Strength training. Single versus multiple sets. *Sports Medicine, 26*(2), 73-84.

Carpinelli, R. N., Otto, R. M., & Winett, R. A. (2004). A critical analysis of the ACSM Position stand on resistance training: insufficient evidence to support recommended training protocols. *Journal of Exercise Physiology online*, *7*(3)1-60.

Ehlenz, H., Grosser, M., & Zimmermann, E. (1998). *Krafttraining. Grundlagen, Methoden, Übungen, Leistungssteuerung, Trainingsprogramme [Strength training. Basics, methods, exercises, performance management, training programs]* (6th ed.). München: BLV Sportwissen.

Feigenbaum, M. S., & Pollock, M. L. (1997). Strength training - rationale for current guidelines for adult fitness programs. *Physician and Sports Medicine, 25*(2), 44-46, 49, 54-56, 63, 64.

Fleck, S. J. (1999). Periodized strength training: a critical review. *Journal of Strength and Conditioning Research, 13*(1), 82-89.

Fröhlich, M., Schmidtbleicher, D., & Emrich, E. (2002). Belastungssteuerung im Muskelaufbautraining. Belastungsnormativ Intensität versus Wiederholungszahl [Training control in hypertrophy training. Intensity vs. repetition]. *Deutsche Zeitschrift für Sportmedizin, 53*(3), 79-83.

Galvao, D. A., & Taaffe, D. R. (2004). Single- vs. multiple-set resistance training: recent developments in the controversy. *Journal of Strength and Conditioning Research, 18*(3), 660-667.

Gearhart, R. E., Goss, F. L., Lagally, K. M., Jakicic, J. M., Gallagher, J., Gallagher, K. I., et al. (2002). Ratings of perceived exertion in active muscle during high-intensity and low-intensity resistance exercise. *Journal of Strength and Conditioning Research, 16*(1), 87-91.

Gießing, J. (2003). Trainingsplanung und -steuerung beim Muskelaufbautraining. Das Konzept vom individuellen hypothetischen Maximalgewicht (h1-RM) als methodische Alternative [Planning and management of training for muscle hypertrophy training. The concept of the individual hypothetical maximum (h1-RM) as a methodological alternative]. *Leistungssport, 33*(4), 26-31.

Glass, S. C., & Stanton, D. R. (2004). Self-selected resistance training intensity in novice weightlifters. *Journal of Strength and Conditioning Research, 18*(2), 324-327.

Haff, G. G. (2004a). Roundtable discussion: Periodization of training part 1. *Strength and Conditioning Journal, 26*(1), 50-69.

Haff, G. G. (2004b). Roundtable discussion: Periodization of training part 2. *Strength and Conditioning Journal, 26*(2), 56-70.

Hoeger, W., Baratte, S., Hale, D., & Hopkins, D. (1987). Relationship between repetitions and selected percentages of one repetition maximum. *Journal of Applied Sport Science Research, 1*(1) 11-13.

Hoeger, W., Baratte, S., Hale, D., & Hopkins, D. (1990). Relationship between repetitions and selected percentages of one repetition maximum: A comparison between untrained and trained males and females. *Journal of Applied Sport Science Research, 4*(2), 47-54.

Hoffman, J. R. (2002). Periodized training for the strength/power athlete. *NSCA´s Performance Training Journal, 1*(9), 8-15.

Kemmler, W., Engelke, K., Lauber, D., Weineck, J., Hensen, J., & Kalender, W. A. (2002). Exercise effects on fitness and BMD in early postmenopausal women: 1 year EFOPS results. *Medicine & Science in Sports & Exercise, 34*(12), 2115-2123.

Kemmler, W., Engelke, K., Lauber, D., Weineck, J., Hensen, J., & Kalender, W. A. (2004). Impact of intense exercise on physical fitness, quality of life, and bone mineral density in early post-menopausal women. Year 2 results of the Erlangen Fitness Osteoporosis Prevention Study (EFOPS). *Archives of Internal Medicine, 164*(1084-1091).

Kemmler, W., Lauber, D., Engelke, K., & Weineck, J. (2004). Effects of single- vs. multiple-set resistance training on maximum strength and body composition in trained postmenopausal women. *Journal of Strength and Conditioning Research, 18*(4), 689-694.

Kemmler, W., Lauber, D., Mayhew, D., & Wassermann, A. (2005). Predicting maximal strength in trained postmenopausal woman. *Journal of Strength and Conditioning Research, submitted*.

Kemmler, W., Lauber, D., von Stengel, S., Weineck, J., Kalender, W. A., & Engelke, K. (2005). Exercise effects on risk factors in early postmenopausal women: 3y EFOPS results. *Medicine & Science in Sports & Exercise, 37*(2), 194-303.

Kemmler, W., Lauber, D., Weineck, J., Mayhew, J., Kalender, W. A., & Engelke, K. (2005). Trainingssteuerung im Gesundheitssport. Lastvorgabe versus subjektive Intensitätswahl im präventivsportlichen Krafttraining [Management of training in health sports. Loading versus subjective intensity in preventive strength training]. *Deutsche Zeitschrift für Sportmedizin, 56*(6), 21-26.

Kenny, R. A., Rubenstein, I. Z., Martin, F. C., & Tinetti, M. E. (2001). Guideline for the prevention of falls in older persons. American Geriatrics Society, British Geriatrics Society, and American Academy of Orthopaedic Surgeons Panel on Falls Prevention. *Journal of the American Geriatrics Society, 49*(5), 664-672.

Kohrt, W. M., Bloomfield, S. A., Little, K. D., Nelson, M. E., & Yingling, V. R. (2004). American College of Sports Medicine Position Stand: physical activity and bone health. *Medicine & Science in Sports & Exercise, 366*(11), 1985-1996.

Kraemer, W. J. (1997). A series of studies - the physiological basis for strength training in American football: fact over philosophy. *Journal of Strength and Conditioning Research, 11*(3), 131-142.

Kraemer, W. J., Gordon, S. E., Fleck, S. J., Marchitelli, L. J., Mello, R., Dziados, J. E., et al. (1991). Endogenous anabolic hormonal and growth factor responses to heavy resistance exercise in males and females. *International Journal of Sports Medicine, 12*(2), 228-235.

Kraemer, W. J., Ratamess, N., Fry, A. C., Triplett-McBride, T., Koziris, L. P., Bauer, J. A., et al. (2000). Influence of resistance training volume and periodization on physiological and performance adaptations in collegiate women tennis players. *The American Journal of Sports Medicine, 28*(5), 626-633.

Kramer, J. B., Stone, M. H., O'Bryant, H. S., Conley, M. S., Johnson, R. L., Nieman, D. C., et al. (1997). Effects of single vs. multiple sets of weight training: impact of volume, intensity, and variation. *Journal of Strength and Conditioning Research, 11*(3), 143-147.

LeSuer, D. A., McCormick, J. H., Mayhew, J. L., Wasserstein, R. L., & Arnold, M. D. (1997). The accuracy of prediction equations for estimating 1-RM performance in the bench press, squat, and deadlift. *Journal of Strength and Conditioning Research, 11*(4), 211-213.

Marcus, R. (1998). Exercise: moving in the right direction. *Journal of Bone and Mineral Research, 13*(12), 1793-1796.

Marschall, F., & Fröhlich, M. (1999). Überprüfung des Zusammenhangs von Maximalkraft und maximaler Wiederholungszahl bei deduzierten submaximalen Intensitäten [Testing the correlation between maximal strength and repetition maximum for deduced lower levels of intensity]. *Deutsche Zeitschrift für Sportmedizin, 50*(10), 311-315.

Marx, J. O., Ratamess, N. A., Nindl, B. C., Gotshalk, L. A., Volek, J. S., Dohi, K., et al. (2001). Low-volume circuit versus high-volume periodized resistance training in women. *Medicine & Science in Sports & Exercise, 33*(4), 635-643.

Mayhew, J. L., Ball, T. E., Busby, K. L., Arnold, M. D., & Bowen, J. C. (1992). Relative muscular endurance performance as a predictor of bench press strength in college men and women. *Journal of Applied Sport Science Research, 6*, 200-206.

Mayhew, J. L., Clemens, J. C., Busky, K. L., Cannon, J. S., Ware, J. S., & Brown, J. C. (1995). Cross-validation of equations to predict 1-RM bench press from repetitions-to-failure. *Medicine & Science in Sports & Exercise, 27*, S209.

Mayhew, J. L., Prinster, J. L., Ware, J. S., Zimmer, D. L., Arabas, J. R., & Bemben, M. G. (1995). Muscular endurance repetitions to predict bench press strength in men of different training levels. *Journal of Sports Medicine and Physical Fitness, 35*(2), 108-113.

Messier, S. P., & Dill, M. E. (1985). Alterations in strength and maximal oxygen uptake consequent to Nautilus circuit weight training. *Research Quarterly for Exercise and Sport, 56*(4), 345-351.

Nicklas, B. J., Ryan, A. J., Treuth, M. M., Harman, S. M., Blackman, M. R., Hurley, B. F., et al. (1995). Testosterone, growth hormone and IGF-I responses to acute and chronic resistive exercise in men aged 55-70 years. *International Journal of Sports Medicine, 16*(7), 445-450.

O´Conner, B., Simmons, J., & O´Shea, P. (1989). *Weigth training today*. St Paul, MN: West Publ.

Pincivero, D. M., Coelho, A. J., & Campy, R. M. (2003). Perceived exertion and maximal quadriceps femoris muscle strength during dynamic knee extension exercise in young adult males and females. *European Journal Applied Physiology, 89*(2), 150-156.

Rhea, M. R., Alvar, B. A., Ball, S. D., & Burkett, L. N. (2002). Three sets of weight training superior to 1 set with equal intensity for eliciting strength. *Journal of Strength and Conditioning Research, 16*(4), 525-529.

Rhea, M. R., Alvar, B. A., Burkett, L. N., & Ball, S. D. (2003). A meta-analysis to determine the dose response for strength development. *Medicine & Science in Sports & Exercise, 35*(3), 456-464.

Rhea, M. R., Ball, S. D., Phillips, W. T., & Burkett, L. N. (2002). A comparison of linear and daily undulating periodized programs with equated volume and intensity for strength. *Journal of Strength and Conditioning Research, 16*(2), 250-255.

Rhea, M. R., Landers, D. M., Alvar, B. A., & Arent, S. M. (2003). The effects of competition and the presence of an audience on weight lifting performance. *Journal of Strength and Conditioning Research, 17*(2), 303-306.

Ryan, A. S., Pratley, R. E., Elahi, D., & Goldberg, A. P. (1995). Resistive training increases fat-free mass and maintains RMR despite weight loss in postmenopausal women. *Journal of Applied Physiology, 79*(3), 818-823.

Sanborn, K., Boros, R., Hruby, J., Schilling, B., O´Bryant, H. S., Johnson, R. L., et al. (2000). Short-term performance effects of weight training with multiple sets not to failure vs. a single set to failure in women. *Journal of Strength and Conditioning Research, 14*(3), 328-331.

Schlumberger, A., Stec, J., & Schmidtbleicher, D. (2001). Single- vs. multiple-set strength training in women. *Journal of Strength and Conditioning Research, 15*(3), 284-289.

Stone, M. H., Johnson, R. L., & Carter, D. R. (1979). A short term comparison of two different methods of resistance training on leg strength and power. *Athletic Training, 14*, 158-160.

Stone, M. H., Potteiger, J. A., Pierce, K. C., Proulx, C. M., O´Bryant, H. S., Johnson, R. L., et al. (2000). Comparison of the effects of three different weight-training programs on the one repetition maximum squat. *Journal of Strength and Conditioning Research, 14*(3), 332-337.

Weineck, J. (2000). *Sportbiologie*. [Biology of sports]. Balingen: Spitta-Verlag.

Wolfe, B. L., LeMura, L. M., & Cole, P. J. (2004). Quantitative analysis of single- vs. multiple-set programs in resistance training. *Journal of Strength and Conditioning Research, 18*(1), 35-47.

Wood, T. M., Maddalozzo, G. F., & Harter, R. A. (2002). Accuracy of seven predictions for predicting 1-RM performance of apparently healthy, sedentary older adults. *Measurement in Physical Education and Exercise Science, 6*(2), 67-94.

MARK BISHOP & THOMAS KAMINSKI

A comparison of enhanced-eccentric resistance training and traditional training for increasing strength

Keywords: overload, eccentric repetition maximum, hamstrings, biceps, quadriceps

Introduction

The primary role of eccentric (lengthening) muscle actions during many daily activities such as walking, and running has been described as one of deceleration and energy absorption (Stauber, 1989). Training regimens that do not contain eccentric actions may not prepare individuals for the eccentric loading that occurs during many athletic and daily activities. Eccentric loading causes damage to the intrinsic muscular mechanisms. Enzymatic markers of muscle damage following exercise are commonly found after performance of eccentric exercise (Ploutz-Snyder, Giamis, Formikell, & Rosenbaum, 2001) and 'preconditioning' a muscle by training with eccentric muscle actions will decrease the damage associated with subsequent bouts of eccentric exercise (Sacco & Jones, 1992; Whitehead, Allen, Morgan, & Proske, 1998).

In addition to recognizing the functional significance of training with eccentric muscle actions, training studies have demonstrated that morphological changes in muscle have been greatest in those studies combining both concentric and eccentric contractions (Colliander & Tesch, 1990; Friedmann et al., 2004; Johnson, Adamansky, Tennoe, & Stromme, 1972). It has been postulated that increases in connective tissue that are associated with eccentric muscle actions contribute to muscular hypertrophy (MacDougall, Sale, Alway, & Sutton, 1984) and larger muscle fibers may resist injury by nature of their size (Stauber, 1989). Eccentric muscle actions have the potential to generate greater muscular forces at lower metabolic cost than concentric muscle actions (LaStayo, Ewy, Pierotti, Johns, & Lindstedt, 2003).

Hamstring injuries are a common and often debilitating occurrence among athletes performing eccentrically demanding maneuvers. Some studies have suggested that poor eccentric hamstring strength is a predisposing element of hamstring injuries in sprinting athletes (Jonhagen, Nemeth, & Eriksson, 1994; Stanton & Purdam, 1989). Studies have indicated that improving eccentric torque production in the hamstring muscles will decrease subsequent muscle strain injuries during a competitive season (Askling, Karlsson, & Thorstensson, 2003).

Eccentric exercise has been shown in some studies to cause strength gains greater than those of concentric training (Brandenburg & Docherty, 2002; Farthing & Chilibeck, 2003; Higbie, Cureton, Warren, & Prior, 1996) while others have not confirmed these results (Dudley, Tesch, Miller, & Buchanan, 1991; Tomberlin et al., 1991). Further studies have shown that a program combining concentric with eccentric contractions is superior to training to with concentric actions only (Dudley et al., 1991; Hortobagyi & Katch, 1990; Kaminski, Wabberson, & Murphy, 1998). It is also well established that eccentric preloading of a muscle improves the power generation of that muscle (Cronin, McNair, & Marshall, 2000; Doan et al., 2002).

When using traditional isotonic strengthening programs, the maximal amount of weight lifted is limited to that developed during the concentric phase. This weight represents a different training load dependent on whether it is compared to the maximal tension developed concentrically, or eccentrically; that is, it is estimated that eccentric muscle actions may generate 140 % of the maximal tension generated by a concentric muscle action. By way of illustration, consider a person who can perform a concentric one repetition maximum lift of 100 kg. This weight represents 100 % of the concentric tension of the muscle but may only be 70 % of the eccentric potential of the muscle.

The development of an isotonic-eccentric device, the Negator™ (Myonics Corporation, Metairie, LA, USA) that allows for enhancement of the eccentric phase, overcomes this limitation without changing the existing variable resistance machinery of strength training apparatuses. By enhancing the eccentric weight, the muscle can be mechanically loaded optimally during both concentric and eccentric phases of a lift. All experiments described in this paper used this technology.

The Negator consists of a separate mechanically controlled weight stack (2.3 kg increments) that attaches to a standard variable resistance device. The device provides assistance during the concentric phase of the lift. When the weight-stack of the strength-training device passes the calibrated location, the Negator™ de-activates, removing the assistance. The effect of removing the resistance is that the entire weight must be lowered. In this manner, the concentric and eccentric load within in the same repetition can be varied and subsequently manipulated independently.

Consider a subject with an arm curl C1-RM of 50 kilograms, and a training protocol that calls for the concentric phase starting weight to be 66 % of 50 kg, and the eccentric phase starting weight to be 100 % of 50 kg. The arm curl machine would be set at 50 kg and the Negator™ activated to provide 16 kg of assistance during the concentric phase (making the concentric weight 34 kg). At the completion of the concentric phase, the Negator™ would deactivate, removing the assistance, and the subject would then lower the entire 50 kg during the eccentric phase.

In this paper, we will present data from several studies that investigate changes in muscular performance after training with enhanced-eccentric muscle actions.

Methods

Subjects

The University Institutional Review Board approved the methods and procedures used in all investigations. Documented informed consent for testing and training was obtained from all participants prior to initial testing. All isometric and isokinetic muscle action testing was done on a Kin Com 125 AP dynamometer (Chattanooga Group, Inc., Chattanooga, TN, USA).

Experimental study (cf. Kaminski et al., 1998)

Given previous evidence that eccentric hamstring training decreased hamstring strain injury during a competitive soccer season, we wanted to examine the response of hamstring muscles to eccentric-enhanced training.

Twenty-seven male students volunteered to participate in Experiment 1 (cf. table 1). All subjects filled out a pre-participation health status questionnaire to determine eligibility. Parameters for inclusion were no previous injuries to the hamstrings, knee and hip joints, no history of performance enhancing drug use, no weight training of the lower extremity during the past 6 months, and no previous illness/condition limiting participation. Subjects were randomly assigned to one of three groups resulting in nine subjects per group (control, enhanced-eccentric, traditional). Lower extremity dominance was determined by asking each participant which leg they would use to kick a ball with.

Table 1. Anthropometric data of subjects within each group in Experiment 1. NEG = concentric/enhanced-eccentric, TRAD = concentric/eccentric, CONT = control group. n = 9 for each group. All values expressed as Mean ± 1SD

	NEG	TRAD	CONT
age (years)	22.9 ± 3.8	23.3 ± 3.5	22.4 ± 1.8
height (cm)	178.2 ± 6.6	176.6 ± 7.5	181.0 ± 7.6
weight (kg)	78.7 ± 6.3	79.4 ± 14.6	87.1 ± 15.4

Test procedures

Subjects reported for C1-RM and isokinetic strength pre-testing on two separate occasions. Each session began by having the subjects perform a three-minute warm-up on a stationary bicycle. Each subject performed a series of lower extremity flexibility exercises including hamstring, quadriceps and calf stretches followed this. Concentric one repetition maximum (C1-RM) data were determined using a Cybex (Cybex Division of Lumex, Inc. Ronkonkoma, NY) isotonic prone hamstring curl apparatus. A standardized C1-RM protocol was used (Wathen, 1994).

Concentric and eccentric peak torque values were obtained at test velocities of 60°/s and 180°/s. Subjects were positioned seated in the dynamometer chair with their body securely fastened to the seat and the thigh held firmly by the thigh stabilizer. Subjects performed 3 submaximal and 3 maximal warm-up repetitions prior to testing at each velocity. A one-minute rest was provided between warm-up and test repetitions. Subjects performed a total of three maximal concentric followed by eccentric repetitions at each velocity. A two-minute rest was provided between velocities. The order of velocity presentation was randomized using a coin flip. Peak torque (Nm) values were derived from the three test repetitions both concentrically and eccentrically.

Training procedures

Subjects assigned to the eccentric and concentric training groups began a six-week hamstring strength-training program. Subjects exercised two times each week for a total of 12 training sessions. Control group subjects refrained from lower extremity strength training during the study. Each workout session began with a 3-minute stationary bicycle warm-up followed by lower extremity flexibility exercises. Each group started with one set of 8 repetitions using 50 % of their C1-RM. The concentric and eccentric load was equal during this warm-up set. Following the warm-up set those subjects in the concentric training group performed two sets of 8 repetitions using a weight equal to 80 % of their C1-RM value. Those subjects in the eccentric training group performed two workout sets of 8 repetitions; however, the concentric load was placed at 40 % of the C1-RM and the eccentric load was placed at 100 % of the C1-RM. A one-minute rest period was given between each set. At the conclusion of each workout session the subjects were asked to assess their perceived level of exertion using the modified Borg scale (Borg, 1978). Training sessions were separated by a two-day rest period.

For subjects who were able to complete both training sets of 8 repetitions without failure, an 'adjusted' C1-RM value was increased by 5.5 kg (12 lb.). The next strengthening workout used this adjusted C1-RM value. The concentric training group therefore maintained a workout load equal to 80 % of their adjusted C1-RM at all times, while the eccentric group maintained a concentric/eccentric load ratio of 40 % and 100 % of their adjusted C1-RM. If progression criteria were not met, the subject would repeat the same workout during the next training session. Each subsequent training session, subjects were asked to report their level of muscle soreness (none, mild, moderate, severe), and whether or not that soreness limited their activities (none, mild, moderate, severe) between training sessions.

In addition to a post-test, each subject completed a post study questionnaire determining compliance, perceived level of progression, muscle soreness, and incidence of low back pain.

Statistical analysis

We used the SPSS for Macintosh Release 6.1.1 (SPSS Inc., Chicago, IL) statistical package to analyze the data. C1-RM/BW (BW = body weight) ratios (kg/kg) and isokinetic peak torque/BW ratios (Nm/kg) served as the dependent measures. Separate mixed model repeated measures ANOVA's were used to determine if any differences existed between the pre and post test conditions among the groups for both dependent measures. The isokinetic PT/BW ratio measures were analyzed utilizing separate ANOVA's for the concentric and eccentric muscle actions at both $60°.s^{-1}$ and $180°.s^{-1}$. Level of muscle soreness was used as the dependent measure to determine if differences in muscle soreness existed between each of the three training groups.

Muscle soreness was assigned a number value to correspond with the participants answer (0 = none, 1 = mild, 2 = moderate, and 3 = severe). A Wilcoxon Rank Sum procedure was utilized to analyze the non-parametric muscle soreness values. An a priori alpha significance level of $p = 0.05$.

Results

The C1-RM/BW ratio ANOVA revealed a significant group by test interaction [$F_{(2, 24)} = 20.20$; $p < 0.001$]. Tukey post hoc tests determined that there were significant differences between the mean C1-RM/BW ratios for pre and post-test measures in the eccentric and concentric training groups. C1-RM/BW ratios improved 28.8 % in the eccentric training group and improved 19.0 % in the concentric training group following 6 weeks of hamstring strength training. There was no notable change in the control group (see figure 1).

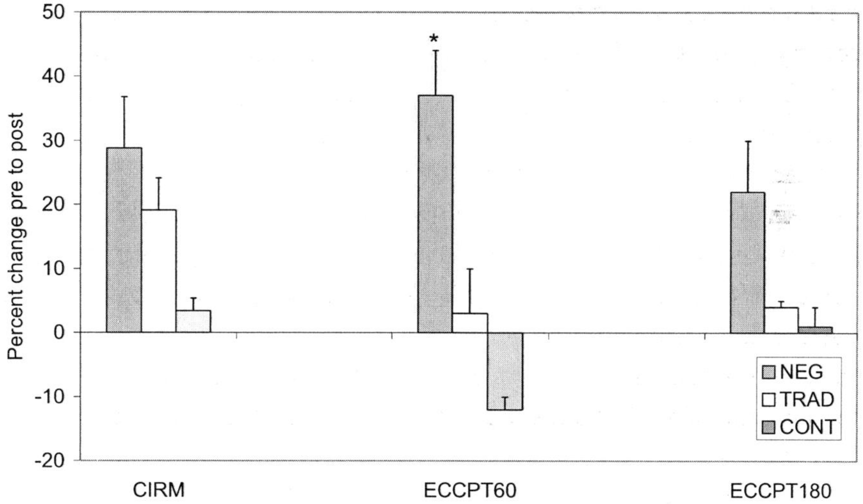

*Figure 1. Percentage change pre-test to post-test. C1-RM – Concentric one repetition maximum, ECCPT60 – peak eccentric torque at 60°/s, ECCPT180 – peak eccentric torque at 180°/s. NEG = concentric/enhanced-eccentric. TRAD = concentric/eccentric. CONT = control. * - NEG significantly different from the other groups (p < 0.05)*

Eccentric isokinetic PT/BW ratios at both 60°/s and 180°/s improved significantly (37.7 % and 22.0 % respectively) from pre to post testing in the eccentric training group only ([$F_{(2, 24)} = 6.11$; $p = 0.007$] and 180°/s [$F_{(2, 24)} = 5.88$; $p = 0.008$]). There were no significant changes in eccentric PT/BW ratios in either the concentric training group or the control group (see figure 1). Interestingly, when the concentric isokinetic PT/BW ratios were analyzed, no interactions occurred between group and test factors [$F_{(2, 24)} = 1.55$; $p = 0.233$] at 60°/s and [$F_{(2, 24)} = 1.35$; $p = 0.279$] at 180°/s. There were some trends that indicated improvements in concentric isokinetic PT/BW ratios in both the eccentric and concentric training groups.

The results of the Wilcoxon Rank Sum procedure indicated that a significant difference in DOMS was evident after day 1 between the groups ($p = 0.012$). Muscle soreness values for the eccentric training group averaged 0.25 ± 0.51, while those in the concentric training group averaged 0.07 ± 0.26. The control group had no soreness. However, no significant differences in DOMS existed between the groups for successive training days.

Our results suggest that an enhanced eccentric strengthening program utilizing eccentric loads equal to the concentric 1-RM can occur twice a week, without being deterred by DOMS. Additionally, traditional training did not improve eccentric isokinetic PT/BW ratios and isotonic concentric and eccentric strength training had little effect on concentric isokinetic PT/BW ratios.

Experimental study 2 (cf. Barstow, Bishop, & Kaminski, 2003)

For Experiment 2, we examined the response of an upper extremity muscle group, elbow flexors, to eccentric-enhanced training. In contrast to Experiment 1, we chose to include subjects only if they had experience in weight training the upper extremity. We chose to do this because of concerns regarding possible effects of heavy eccentric load on the long head of biceps and the attachment to the glenoid labrum. Thirty-nine subjects (eight males, 31 females) volunteered for Experiment 2. Subjects were included if they had weight-trained their upper extremities twice a week for at least three months. Current musculoskeletal pathology affecting the upper extremity, any medical limitations to their exercise, or a history of anabolic steroid use resulted in exclusion from the study. Subject data are summarized in table 2.

Table 2. Anthropometric data of subjects within each group in Experiment 2. NEG = concentric/enhanced-eccentric, TRAD = concentric/eccentric, CONT = control group. n = 13 for each group. All values expressed as Mean ± 1SD

	NEG	TRAD	CONT
age (years)	23.6 ± 5.2	22.3 ± 0.8	20.6 ± 1.0
height (cm)	167.0 ± 9.4	167.0 ± 9.0	168.7 ± 6.7
weight (kg)	62.4 ± 14.1	64.8 ± 6.7	72.4 ± 12.3
strength index ($N \cdot kg^{-1}$)	1.1 ± 0.3	1.0 ± 0.3	1.1 ± 0.3

For this experiment we tested subjects across three modes of muscle action: isometric, isokinetic and isotonic. During isometric and isokinetic testing, the subject sat upright on the dynamometer seat in the standard position for testing of elbow flexion described by the manufacturer. The subject was encouraged to give a maximal effort during all muscle actions and received both visual and verbal feedback to maximize contraction effort (McNair & Stanley,

1996). The same evaluator tested all subjects and remained blinded to subject group over the course of the investigation. All subjects completed a practice and familiarization session.

Peak isometric force was measured at five angles of elbow flexion (10°, 25°, 60°, 85°, and 110°) on the right upper extremity. The order of testing was counter-balanced using a latin square. Peak isometric force was measured three times at each joint angle, and then averaged to provide one force value for each angle tested. There was twenty seconds of rest given between each trial at the same angle and three minutes of rest between each testing angle (Kaminski & Hartsell, 2002). A sub-group of six subjects returned within another five days to repeat testing to determine reliability of the isometric test procedure.

Isokinetic testing was performed at 40°/s. This was based on the time taken by the subject when training isotonicly. A warm-up of 10 submaximal repetitions was done, followed by three minutes of rest. Each subject performed three repetitions of maximal concentric and eccentric elbow flexion actions. One minute of rest was given between muscle actions. All subjects verbally indicated that they had given a maximal effort during both testing procedure using a modified perceived exertion scale (Borg, 1978).

C1-RM was determined by sequential one-repetition bilateral arm curls with increasing resistance on the Cybex arm curl machine (Cybex, Division of Lumex, Ronkonkoma, NY).

Resistance training

After all subjects had completed their initial strength tests, isometric force was averaged across all joint angles and expressed relative to body weight (Newton x kg^{-1}). Subjects were then rank-ordered based on this strength index value. Following this, the group assignment for the first subject was randomly drawn from the first row of a latin square. Subsequent subjects were placed in one of the concentric-enhanced eccentric group (NEG), the concentric-eccentric group (TRAD), or a control group (CONT) using a latin square based on the first assignment. The control group continued habitual activity without modification to their training regimen. All training was done using the Cybex arm curl machine. The seat height of the arm curl machine was adjusted so that the subject's right arm was maintained in 70° of glenohumeral joint flexion when resting on the elbow pad. Subjects performed a two-handed arm curl on a 'two count' (two seconds up for the concentric phase and two seconds down for the eccentric phase). This was chosen since it represented the manner in which student athletes at the University are instructed to move their forearm during resistance exercise using free weights. Subjects in the TRAD group began training at 60 % C1-RM.

If subjects could perform all the required repetitions at the prescribed resistance, training weight was increased 5 % at the next training session. As long as the subjects could maintain a minimum of 66 % of the asked repetitions, the new weight was maintained as the training weight for subsequent sessions, otherwise the weight was decreased by approximately 5 %. Once subjects were able to perform 100 % of all the required repetitions at the new weight, it was again increased 5 %. The NEG group used the same training protocols and starting concentric weight (60 % C1-RM) as the traditional group. The eccentric weight, however, began at 100 % C1-RM. The load progression regimen was applied to both the concentric and eccentric training weights subjects trained twice a week for twelve weeks. Regular telephone calls were used to ensure subject compliance.

A one-way ANOVA was used to compare each anthropometric variable among groups before training. The test-retest reliability of the isometric testing protocol was determined using an intraclass correlation coefficient ($ICC_{2,1}$) with the isometric strength index as the dependent variable. Changes in C1-RM were identified using a mixed model (between = group, pre and post-test = within) repeated-measures ANOVA. The dependent variable for isometric testing was the percent change in the mean peak isometric force at each testing angle. Training effects were determined using a mixed model ANOVA (between = group, within = angle) with post-hoc one-way ANOVA contrasts and follow up pairwise comparisons using Dunn-Bonferroni corrections.

There were multiple variables assessed for isokinetic testing: peak concentric and eccentric force, and average concentric and eccentric force. Given the close association between these dependent variables, a multivariate analysis of variance (MANOVA) was conducted with one-way post-hoc contrasts performed, followed by pairwise comparisons using Dunn-Bonferroni corrections. The family-wise type 1 error was set at 5 %.

Results

There were no differences noted among the groups for any of the anthropometric data assessed. Test-retest reliability of the isometric strength index was found to be high (ICC = 0.94).

C1-RM

Training load increased an average of 27 % over the course of the twelve-week training period. After 24 training sessions, NEG group increased elbow flexion C1-RM by 15.5 %, and TRAD by 13.8 %.
Despite these changes, no significant interactions were noted between group and time ($F_{(2, 76)} = 1.2$; $p = 0.44$) for C1-RM, nor were any group main effects apparent ($F_{(2, 37)} = 0.51$; $p = 0.48$). There was a trend for NEG to have increased C1-RM greater than CONT but this difference did not reach significance and there were no differences between NEG and TRAD training regimens. However, twelve weeks of training did result in a significant increase in C1-RM ($F_{(1, 36)} = 20.0$; $p < 0.05$) for the training groups.

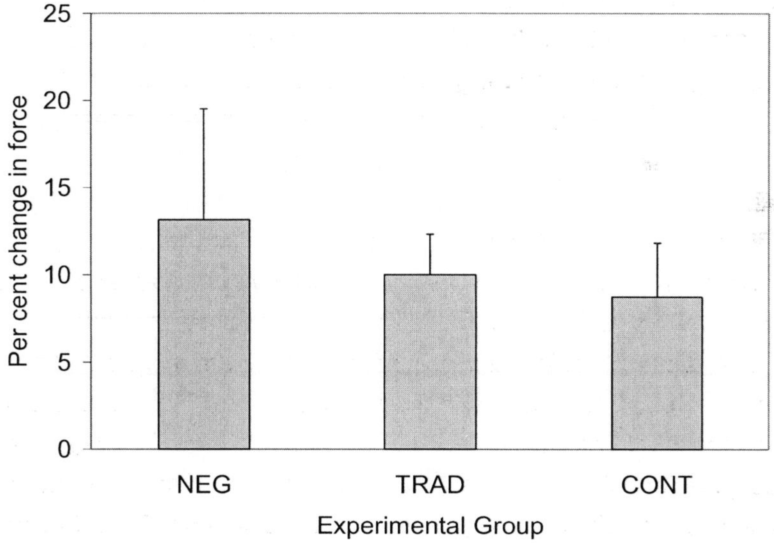

Figure 2. Percent change (pre- to post) in concentric one-repetition-maximum of the biceps brachii in Experimental Study 2. Bars represent 1 SEM. NEG = concentric/enhanced-eccentric. TRAD = concentric/eccentric. CONT = control

Isometric force

No interaction was noted among the groups at any of the isometric angles tested ($F_{(7, 28)} = 1.48$; $p = 0.17$). One subject in the NEG group improved at

110° by 150 % resulting in the large amount of variability within the NEG group (the average difference in isometric force produced at 110° for the group was 36.5 ± 23.1 %). After 12 weeks of strength training, there was no group main effect ($F_{(2, 32)} = 0.15$; $p = 0.86$) indicating that the training groups were not different statistically from the control group. However, there was a main effect for 'angle' ($F_{(4, 108)} = 2.657$; $p = 0.037$). The change in force at 110° was greater than that at 10° ($F_{(1, 29)} = 4.59$; $p = 0.041$) and 85° ($F_{(1, 29)} = 5.56$; $p = 0.025$).

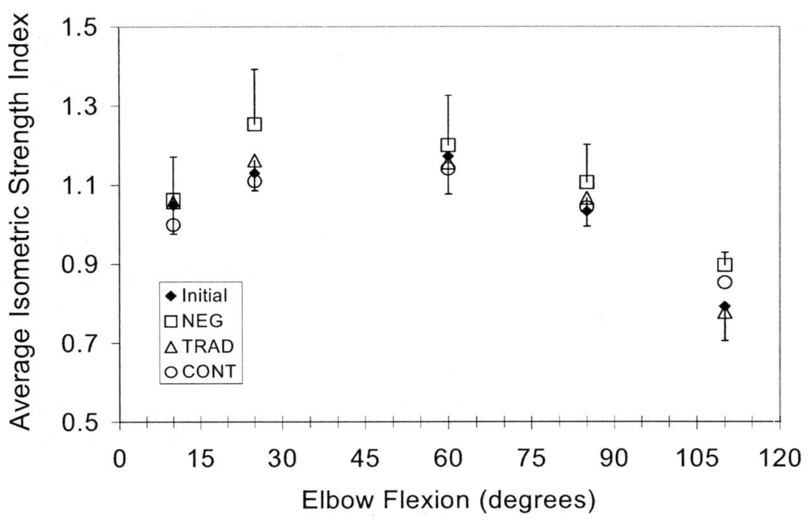

Figure 3. Percent change in isometric force (N) from pre-test to post-test by group. NEG = concentric/enhanced-eccentric, TRAD = concentric/eccentric, CONT = control group. Bars represent 1 SEM. NEG = concentric/enhanced-eccentric. TRAD = concentric/eccentric. CONT = control

Isokinetic force

The MANOVA results (Wilk's Lambda = 0.511; $F_{(8, 38)} = 1.892$; $p = 0.09$) indicated weak evidence of a difference among groups. For example, large percentage changes occurred within the NEG and TRAD groups when considering the average concentric force produced throughout the range of elbow flexion. However, high within group variability resulted in few of these changes being different from zero. Perhaps the most interesting change in isokinetic results was that, on average, the control group showed a decrement in ability to generate peak eccentric torque while the training groups improved.

Perceived exertion (Borg, 1978) was recorded after each set during the training phase of this study. Inspection of the training logs showed that subjects in the NEG group reported a perceived exertion of 9 or 10 on a ten-point scale after each set of exercise. Those in the TRAD group did not report this until the final set of each training session; that is, subjects training in the enhanced-eccentric groups perceived their exertion to be high throughout the entire workout session. Although changes were noted in mean values of C1-RM, and isokinetic variables for the training groups, the within group variability was large. This was a trained pool of subjects and therefore may not have made as much change as might be expected of untrained subjects (Higbie et al., 1996). With this in mind, we had expected that any changes made in trained subjects would be small, however, our a priori power analysis had indicated that, at least on isometric testing, 12 subjects were needed for our effect size to produce statistically significant results. It is apparent that this was not the case.

Experimental study 3 (cf. Levy et al., 2001)

Experiment 3 was developed to assess whether different repetition schemes affected any strength gains made using eccentric-enhanced exercise. Sixteen subjects (age: 22.3 ± 2.6 years; height = 168.1 ± 9.0 cm; weight = 69.6 ± 13.6 kg) volunteered to participate in the 6-week strength training program. Anthropometric data are presented in table 3.

Table 3. Anthropometric data of subjects within each group in Experiment 3. NEG = concentric/enhanced-eccentric, TRAD = concentric/eccentric, CONT = control group. n = 8 for each group. All values expressed as Mean ± 1SD

	low	high
age (years)	22.4 ± 1.1	22.1 ± 0.5
height (cm)	170.0 ± 2.8	166.3 ± 3.3
weight (kg)	75.4 ± 4.8	63.8 ± 4.1

Pre and post-test measurements were taken of thigh girth and C1-RM knee extension strength. Isometric knee extension peak torque (PT) at 5°, 45°, and 75° angles, and isokinetic knee extension PT at 60°/s and 180°/s were tested. Isokinetic testing assessed both eccentric (ECC) and concentric (CON) strength. Subjects were rank ordered according to strength index (see Experiment 2) and randomly assigned into one of the training groups (5 - 7 reps and 15 - 17 reps). Both groups performed enhanced eccentric unilateral knee extension exercises with the dominant leg. Each subject trained one set, twice a week. Each of the five different dependent variables (girth, C1-RM, CON PT, ECC PT and isometric PT) was analyzed using a separate mixed model ANOVA (group = between, time = within) to determine if differences existed between the two training schemes.

Results

Girth

The results of the analysis demonstrated a significant test by dominance interaction [$F_{(1, 14)} = 23.9$; $p < .0001$]. The training leg post-test girth measurement was significantly greater than the pre-test girth measurements (44.93 cm > 43.92 cm).

C1-RM measurements

The results of the analysis demonstrated a significant test by dominance interaction [$F_{(1, 14)} = 15.8$; $p = .001$]. There were no significant differences between the two training groups [$F_{(1, 14)} = .21$; $p = .654$.]

The training leg post-test C1-RM measurements were significantly greater than the pre-test 1-RM measurements (68.32 kg > 60.09 kg). As expected, the post-test dominant 1-RM measurements were significantly greater than both the pre and post-test non-dominant 1-RM measurements. The post-test 1-RM strength measurements in the non-dominant leg were significantly greater than the pre-test 1-RM values (60.09 kg > 57.39 kg).

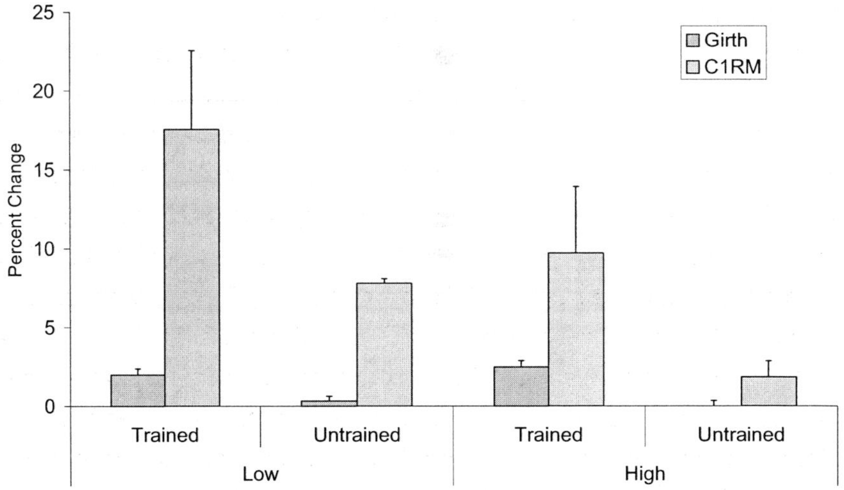

Figure 4. Group effects from Experiment 3. Percent change in thigh girth and concentric one-repetition- maximum (C1-RM) leg extension exercise. Trained – that limb which performed the training, untrained - the limb not trained. High and low refer to the repetition regimen performed during training. Please note that the significant effects were main effects only; that is, the average percent change in the trained limb was greater than the non-trained limb

Eccentric isokinetic strength measurements

The 5 - 7-RM group increased significantly from pre (148.17 Nm) to post (198.81 Nm) testing on the dominant (training) side. It is important to remember that these values contain eccentric isokinetic strength values across both speeds tested (60°/s and 180°/s). Additionally, the 5 - 7-RM group had significantly higher eccentric isokinetic strength values post-test than the 15 - 17-RM group (198.81 Nm > 160.51 Nm). Although there were no differences between the groups, significant increases over time were found for thigh girth, C1-RM, CON PT and isometric PT existed. Interestingly, significant strength increases were also observed in the untrained limb in both groups for the C1-RM test.

Discussion

In Experiment 2, even though training load increased by about 27 % for both training groups, C1-RM results did not support the superiority of enhance-eccentric training to improve isotonic strength in trained subjects. This is in direct contrast to Experiment 1 (Kaminski et al., 1998). In that study, we showed that the enhanced-eccentric group improved C1-RM by 29 % while the traditional group improved 19 % after 6 weeks of training.

We speculate that there are two primary reasons to explain the difference between these two experimental studies. First, the possibility is present that a group difference may have occurred in Experiment 2 at 6 weeks; that is a difference between the eccentric-enhanced training and the traditional training, but this difference then disappeared over the course of the subsequent 6 weeks of training. Previous studies report increased neural adaptation from eccentric training (Aagaard et al., 2000; Hortobagyi, Devita, Money, & Barrier, 2001; Housh, Housh, Weir, & Weir, 1996; Uh, Beynnon, Helie, Alosa, & Renstrom, 2000). Hortobagyi et al. (2001), for example, indicated that in untrained individuals, eccentric overload resulted in improvements in activation of the quadriceps muscle that paralleled increases in peak torque production. Also, we noted in Experiment 3, that significant C1-RM gains were made in the untrained leg.

Previously, we have reported that there appear to be differing activation strategies for controlling concentric and eccentric muscle actions (Bishop, Trimble, Bauer, & Kaminski, 2000). An observation made during training for Experiment 2 was that subjects in the Negator group progressed either the concentric training weight, or the eccentric training weight but rarely both simultaneously. This observation lends credence to the notion that eccentric and concentric muscle actions may have differing time courses to neural adaptation.

Second, our group of trained individuals in Experiment 2 may have reached a ceiling effect regarding improvements in muscle activation and strength gain. Experiment 1 tested novice strength trainers in whom greater gains would be expected.

Also in contrast to Experiment 1, changes in isokinetic torque production were not different among groups in Experiment 2. Subjects trained their elbow flexors with the humerus supported at 70° of shoulder flexion bilaterally, while gripping the Cybex arm curl handle, whereas they were tested using a unilateral forearm flexion protocol with the arm at their side. Winters and Kleweno (1993) examined the effect of shoulder position on torque generation of the elbow flexor muscles. They found significant strength gains in the training position and little or no gains in an unfamiliar position. The presence of a two joint muscle allows for creation of a non-specific angle of testing to be used.

The position of the arm in relation to the thorax alters the length of the long head of biceps and introduces the factor of muscle length specificity. Also the humerus was not supported during testing while it was during training. During testing, therefore, subjects had to dynamically stabilize the trunk and gleno-humeral-scapulothoracic joint complex perhaps resulting in a decreased ability of the prime movers (biceps brachii and brachialis) to generate elbow flexion torque. This is likewise the case for Experiment 1, in which subjects tested with the hip at 90° of flexion but trained with the hip extended, adding an element of angle specificity to the training process. Research into the area of specificity has considered angle, velocity and mode specificity (Morrissey, Harman, & Johnson, 1995). Many researchers have therefore incorporated some elements of mode, angle or velocity specificity into their testing. This may explain the small, but significant carryover seen in their results. By considering posture and two-joint specificity in the development of the non-specific test, this study may have eliminated the carryover seen in other studies. Also it should be considered that a review of blinded versus nonblinded trials demonstrated that when a study is blinded such as the present study, the null hypothesis is likely to prevail.

Results from Experiment 3, appear to indicate that lower repetition schemes with greater load provided improved gains in eccentric peak torque from enhanced-eccentric training. Similar results have been reported more recently that support our finding and indicate that fewer repetitions may be required to maximize adaptation when training with enhanced-eccentric muscle actions. This bodes well when considering rehabilitation applications of enhanced-eccentric training. LaStayo et al. (2003) have demonstrated that older adults with cardiopulmonary conditions can make significant functional gain when training with eccentric overload, at reduced metabolic cost. Patients maybe able to train to improve muscular performance more effectively while placing less stress on the cardiovascular system.

Conclusion

Subjects in all three studies routinely performed strength training with increased loading of eccentric phases motion beyond that expected in traditional training programs. Although subjects did experience DOMS after the first training sessions, these sensations rapidly decreased and did not interfere with the training regimen. Additionally, in Experiment 2, subjects trained for three months with heavy eccentric loads.

Despite this, we had no athlete experience an adverse event, such as a muscular strain, that necessitated withdrawal from the experiment. We believe that our results lend credence to the notion that enhanced-eccentric training can be done safely. This is important in light of recent literature supports the use of enhanced-eccentric training in novice strength trainers, rehabilitation of tendon injuries and older adults and patients.

Although training loads and perceived exertion were greater in the enhanced-eccentric training groups, no clear superiority was noted in the measures we used to assess outcome in Experiments 1 and 2. However, on average, gains were always greater for the enhanced-eccentric training groups, but not statistically different from those gains made in the traditional group. We were predominantly examining group differences. Experiment 2 used groups of trained athletes, in whom the potential for improvement may have reached a ceiling effect. However, some of the improvements made represented gains in personal best lifts for several members of the training groups representing meaningful strength gain, if not statistically significant change. So, although we did not conclude that the enhanced-training program provided superior results, we did find that enhanced-eccentric training improved eccentric peak torque production in the leg, did not cause any adverse injury, was tolerated by all subjects, and increased perceived exertion while training.

Acknowledgements

We would like to thank all the other individuals that participated in these studies as subjects, evaluators or trainers. Special thanks go to Mike MacMillan, M.D, Ian Barstow PT, CSCS and Ethan Levy, MS, CSCS, and Ron Hardouin for engineering assistance and troubleshooting.

References

Aagaard, P., Simonsen, E. B., Andersen, J. L., Magnusson, S. P., Halkjaer-Kristensen, J., & Dyhre-Poulsen, P. (2000). Neural inhibition during maximal eccentric and concentric quadriceps contraction: effects of resistance training. *Journal of Applied Physiology, 89*(6), 2249-2257.

Askling, C., Karlsson, J., & Thorstensson, A. (2003). Hamstring injury occurrence in elite soccer players after preseason strength training with eccentric overload. *Scandinavian Journal of Medicine and Science in Sports, 13*(4), 244-250.

Barstow, I. K., Bishop, M. D., & Kaminski, T. W. (2003). Is enhanced-eccentric resistance training superior to traditional training for increasing elbow flexor strength. *Journal of Sports Science and Medicine, 2*(2), 62-69.

Bishop, M. D., Trimble, M. H., Bauer, J. A., & Kaminski, T. W. (2000). Differential control during maximal concentric and eccentric loading revealed by characteristics of the electromyogram. *Journal of Electromyography and Kinesiology, 10*(6), 399-405.

Borg, G. (1978). Subjective effort in relation to physical performance and working capacity. In H. Pick (Ed.), *Psychology. From Research to Practice.* (pp. 333-361). New York: Plenum Publishing.

Brandenburg, J. P., & Docherty, D. (2002). The effects of accentuated eccentric loading on strength, muscle hypertrophy, and neural adaptations in trained individuals. *Journal of Strength and Conditioning Research, 16*(1), 25-32.

Colliander, E. B., & Tesch, P. A. (1990). Effects of eccentric and concentric muscle actions in resistance training. *Acta Physiologica Scandinavica, 140*(1), 31-39.

Cronin, N., McNair, P. J., & Marshall, R. N. (2000). The role of maximal strength and load on initial power production. *Medicine & Science in Sports & Exercise, 32*(10), 1763-1769.

Doan, B. K., Newton, R. U., Marsit, J. L., Triplett-McBride, N. T., Koziris, L. P., Fry, A. C., et al. (2002). Effects of increased eccentric loading on bench press 1-RM. *Journal of Strength and Conditioning Research, 16*(1), 9-13.

Dudley, G. A., Tesch, P. A., Miller, B. J., & Buchanan, P. (1991). Importance of eccentric actions in performance adaptations to resistance training. *Aviation, Space & Environmental Medicine, 62*(6), 543-550.

Farthing, J. P., & Chilibeck, P. D. (2003). The effect of eccentric training at different velocities on cross-education. *European Journal of Applied Physiology, 89*(6), 570-577.

Friedmann, B., Kinscherf, R., Vorwald, S., Muller, H., Kucera, K., Borisch, S., et al. (2004). Muscular adaptations to computer-guided strength training with eccentric overload. *Acta Physiologica Scandinavica, 182*(1), 77-88.

Higbie, E. J., Cureton, K. J., Warren, G. L., 3rd, & Prior, B. M. (1996). Effects of concentric and eccentric training on muscle strength, cross-sectional area, and neural activation. *Journal of Applied Physiology, 81*(5), 2173-2181.

Hortobagyi, T., Devita, P., Money, J., & Barrier, J. (2001). Effects of standard and eccentric overload strength training in young women. *Medicine & Science in Sports & Exercise, 33*(7), 1206-1212.

Hortobagyi, T., & Katch, F. I. (1990). Role of concentric force in limiting improvement in muscular strength. *Journal of Applied Physiology, 68*(2), 650-658.

Housh, T. J., Housh, D. J., Weir, J. P., & Weir, L. L. (1996). Effects of eccentric-only resistance training and detraining. *International Journal of Sports Science, 17*(2), 145-148.

Johnson, B., Adamansky, K., Tennoe, K., & Stromme, S. (1972). A comparison of concentric and eccentric muscle training. *Medicine & Science in Sports, 4*(8), 35-38.

Jonhagen, B., Nemeth, G., & Eriksson, E. (1994). Hamstring injuries in sprinters - The role of concentric and eccentric hamstring muscle strength and flexibility. *American Journal of Sports Medicine, 22*, 262-266.

Kaminski, T. W., & Hartsell, H. D. (2002). Factors contributing to chronic ankle instability: A strength perspective. *Journal of Athletic Training, 37*(4), 394-405.

Kaminski, T. W., Wabberson, C. V., & Murphy, R. M. (1998). Concentric vs. eccentric hamstring strength training: clinical implications. *Journal of Athletic Training, 33*, 216-221.

LaStayo, P. C., Ewy, G. A., Pierotti, D. D., Johns, R. K., & Lindstedt, S. (2003). The positive effects of negative work: increased muscle strength and decreased fall risk in a frail elderly population. *Journals of Gerontology Series A: Biological Sciences and Medical Sciences, 58*(5), M419-424.

Levy, E. T., Kaminski, T. W., Del Rossi, G., Powers, M. E., Horodyski, M. B., & Dodd, S. L. (2001). Eccentric repetition variation on quadriceps strength and thigh girth. *Journal of Athletic Training, 36*(2), S57.

MacDougall, J. D., Sale, D. G., Alway, S. E., & Sutton, J. R. (1984). Muscle fiber number in biceps brachii in bodybuilders and control subjects. *Journal of Applied Physiology, 57*(5), 1399-1403.

McNair, P. D., J. / Stanley, S. (1996). Verbal encouragement: effects on maximum effort voluntary muscle contraction. *British Journal of Sports Exercise, 27*, 648-660.

Morrissey, M. C., Harman, E. A., & Johnson, M. J. (1995). Resistance training modes: specificity and effectiveness. *Medicine & Science in Sports & Exercise, 27*(5), 648-660.

Ploutz-Snyder, L. L., Giamis, E. L., Formikell, M., & Rosenbaum, A. E. (2001). Resistance training reduces susceptibility to eccentric exercise-induced muscle dysfunction in older women. *Journals of Gerontology Series A: Biological Sciences and Medical Sciences, 56*(9), B384-390.

Sacco, P., & Jones, D. A. (1992). The protective effect of damaging eccentric exercise against repeated bouts of exercise in the mouse tibialis anterior muscle. *Experimental Physiology, 77*(5), 757-760.

Stanton, P., & Purdam, C. (1989). Hamstring injuries in sprinting - The role of eccentric exercise. *Journal of Orthopadic Sports and Phsysiological Therapy, 10*, 343-349.

Stauber, W. T. (1989). Eccentric action of muscles: physiology, injury, and adaptation. *Exercise and Sport Sciences Reviews, 17*, 157-185.

Tomberlin, J. P., Bastford, J. R., Schwen, E., Orte, P., Scott, S., Laughman, R., et al. (1991). Comparative study of isokinetic eccentric and concentric quadriceps training. *Journal of Orthopedic and Sports Physical Therapy, 14*, 31-36.

Uh, B. S., Beynnon, B. D., Helie, B. V., Alosa, D. M., & Renstrom, P. A. (2000). The benefit of a single-leg strength training program for the muscles around the untrained amkle. *American Journal of Sports Medicine, 28*, 568-573.

Wathen, D. (1994). Load assignment. In T. R. Baechle (Ed.), *Essentials of strength training and conditioning* (pp. 435-446). Champaign, IL: Human Kinetics.

Whitehead, N. P., Allen, T. J., Morgan, D. L., & Proske, U. (1998). Damage to human muscle from eccentric exercise after training with concentric exercise. *Journal of Physiology, 512*, 615-620.

Winters, J., & Kleweno, D. (1993). Effects of initial upper-limb alignment on muscle contributions to isometric strength curves. *Journal of Biomechanic, 26*, 143-153.

ANDREAS STRACK & CHRISTOPH EIFLER

The individual lifting performance method (ILP) - a practical method for fitness- and recreational strength training

Keywords: individual lifting performance method, strength training, fitness, prediction, periodized training

Introduction

The individual lifting performance method (ILP) was initially based on practical experiences and has constantly been improved according to current findings. ILP-training is not only applied in fitness training (cf. Strack, 1998a, 1998b, 1999) but also in related contexts like physical therapy (cf. Kempf & Strack, 2001; Strack, 2000).

An overview of ILP is given in table 1. The concept of ILP is based on using submaximal strength tests and adjusting all training parameters on a trainee's current strength level (RM-test, cf. De Lorme, 1945), this test is called "the individual lifting performance test" (ILP-test). Using submaximal strength tests in order to determine an individual's current strength level is an approach that is supported by recent results of strength training research (cf. Buskies & Boeckh-Behrens, 1999; Fröhlich, 2003; Gießing, 2004; Marschall & Fröhlich, 1999).

Table 1: An overview of the training method "individual lifting performance" (ILP) ([1] Percentages of intensity refer to the results of the submaximal tests)

training level	lifting experience (months)	training system	frequency per week	exercises per muscle	sets	repetitions	intensity[1]
orientation stage	0 - 1,5	whole body exercise	1 - 2	1 - 2	1 - 2	10 - 15	trial and error
beginners	> 1,5 - 6	whole body exercise	2	1 - 2	1 - 2	specific	50 - 70%
moderately advanced	> 6 - 12	whole body exercise/split program	2 - 3	2	2	specific	60 - 80 %
advanced	> 12 - 36	whole body exercise/split program	3 - 4	2 - 3	2 - 3	specific	70 - 90 %
elite	> 36	whole body exercise/split program	4 - 6	2 - 4	3 - 4	specific	80 - 100 %

Considering the contradictory recommendations concerning the relationship between work load and number of repetitions depending on specific training goals (cf. Buskies & Boeckh-Behrens, 1999; Fleck & Kraemer, 2004; Fröhlich, 2003; Hoeger, Barette, Hale, & Hopkins, 1987; Hoeger, Hopkins, Barette, & Hale, 1990), the ILP method is based on the following repetition/TUT (time under tension) scheme :

a) strength endurance training: 15 - 30 repetitions, alternatively: a TUT of 50 - 90 seconds (cf. Fröhlich, Klein, Emrich, & Schmidtbleicher, 2001),
b) muscle hypertrophy training: 8 - 15 repetitions, alternatively: a TUT of 20 - 50 seconds,
c) strength training: 5 - 8 repetitions, alternatively: a TUT of < 20 seconds. (Since the ILP method was primarily developed for recreational and fitness training the number of repetitions should be higher than the one to three/five repetitions usually recommended for strength training. Despite this modification strength increases and adaptations on a neuromuscular level can be expected (cf. Fukunaga, 1976; Komi, 1986; MacDougall, Elder, Sale, Moroz, & Sutton, 1980; Pette, 1999).

Applying the ILP method in practical training

The application of the ILP method in practical training is made a lot more convenient by using a special kind of computer software (cf. figure 1 - 3). Training programs based on the ILP method are planned by developing a macrocycle that covers a timescale of six months (see figure 1). The length of the mesocycles depends on the trainee's individual level of performance and lasts between four and twelve weeks. Generally speaking, training cycles which put an emphasis on training volume should be longer than those emphasizing training intensity (cf. Denner, 1998).

Periodization is a decisive factor for continuing progress in strength training. Periodized programs are usually superior to non-periodized training programs (cf. Fleck, 2002; Fleck & Kraemer, 2004). Therefore, training parameters as well as the exercises used are changed for each mesocycle (see figure 2).

Submaximal strength tests are done at the beginning of each new mesocycle. Based on these tests the work loads that are to be used on the various exercises during the new mesocycle are determined. The percentage of maximum training intensity is changed on a weekly basis, regardless of the specific training goal that is emphasised during that particular mesocycle. E. g. moderately advanced trainees, will use 60 to 80 % of the weights they were able to use in the ILP test. Each week 5 % are added (see figure 3). This procedure is the same for all mesocycles and does not depend on the question whether the particular mesocycle focuses on strength, hypertrophy or strength endurance. Increasing training intensity can be achieved by either increasing the number of repetitions or - if that particular mesocycle requires the athlete to do a certain number of repetitions, work load will be increased accordingly.

During the cycle that emphasizes strength endurance, e.g. repetitions will be in the range of 15 to 30. This means that the same number of repetitions is done on all exercises or repetitions are varied from exercise to exercise (15 repetitions for the fist exercise, 20 repetitions for the second one, 25 repetitions for the third one, 30 repetitions for the fourth one).

In order to progressively induce improvements, trainees should go on with the next mesocycle after successfully completing one cycle. This progression makes sure that there is the required progression concerning the three main training parameters (Schlumberger & Schmidtbleicher, 1999). For trainees who intend to keep their present condition and are not necessarily interested in improvements (e.g. when concentrating on a different aspect of their training when strength training is used to supplement the general training program) changing these parameters is not required.

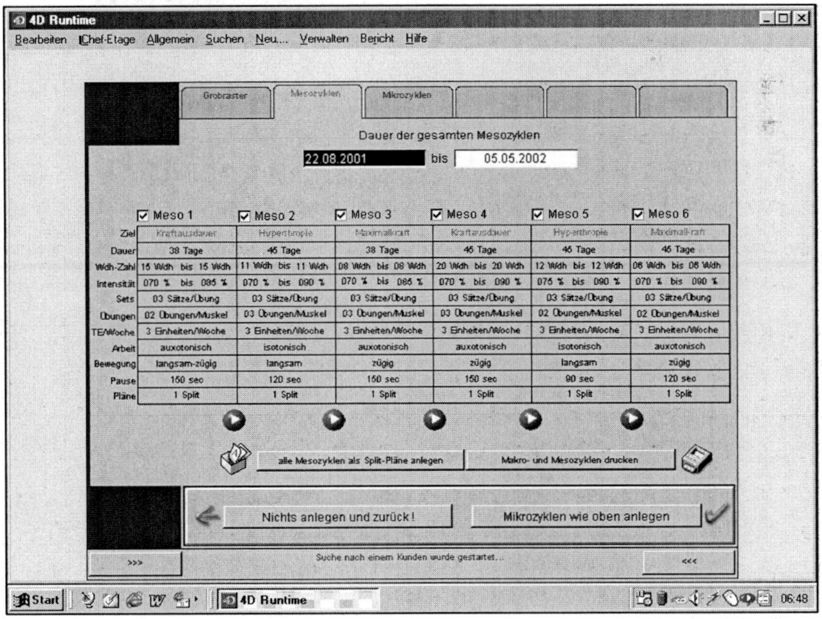

Figure 1: Operating for marcocycle planning (Software by Optifit 2.0; Company Bikom Optifit)

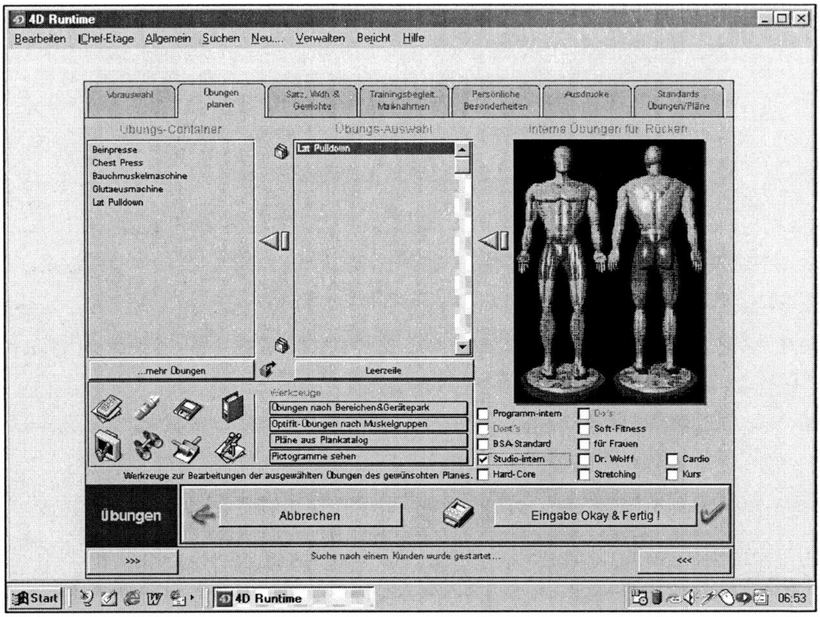

Figure 2: Operating for exercise planning (Software by Optifit 2.0; Company Bikom Optifit)

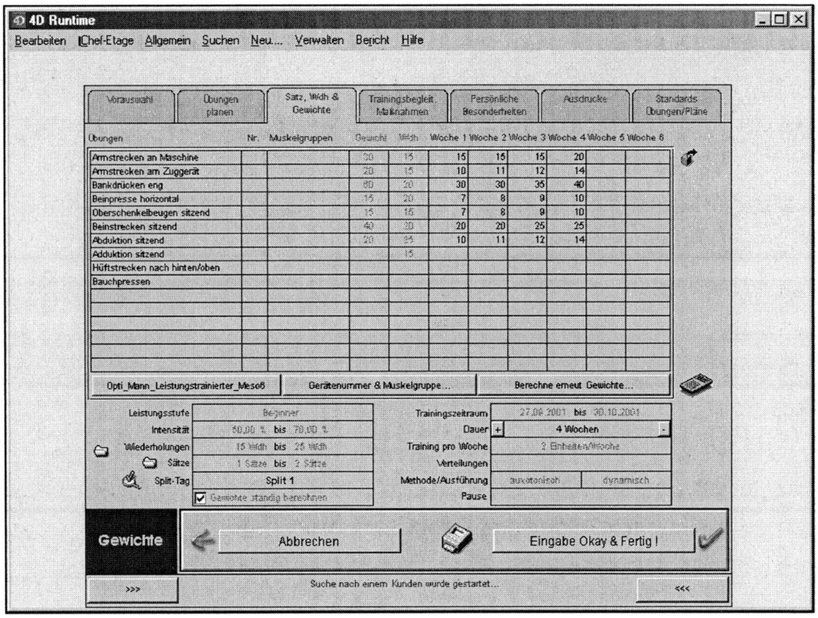

Figure 3: Operating for mesocycle planning (Software by Optifit 2.0; Company Bikom Optifit)

Methods

Subjects

This study was conducted as diplomathesis in the context of attaining the degree „Diplom-Sportlehrer“ at the Universität des Saarlandes (cf. Eifler, 2000). Subjects were two groups of eight students each. The first group consisted of eight beginners (three females and five males) whereas the second group consisted of eight advanced male students who had been strength training for at least one year.

Table 2: Anthropometric data of the subjects

	mean	SD	minimum	maximum
age [yrs]	25.8	2.5	23	33
weight [kg]	73.9	6.9	63	88
height [cm]	179.2	5.3	170	186

Conceptual formulation

Exercises chosen for this study were bench presses on a smith machine and horizontal leg presses. These exercises were chosen because they stress several muscles and training results can be compared to the results of earlier studies (cf. Kraemer & Fry, 1995).

The actual study was preceded by two weeks during which subjects performed two exercises per week doing three sets of 12 repetitions each using 20 % of their bodyweight for bench presses and 50 % of their bodyweight for leg presses. After these two weeks each subject performed a submaximal ILP test doing 12-RM (see tables 2 - 5). Each test set was taken to the point of momentary muscular failure (PMF). In addition to these submaximal ILP tests, the subjects‘ RPE was noted (cf. Borg, 2004).

After these initial tests each subject performed two training sessions per week for six weeks doing three sets of 12 repetitions of each exercise. Training intensity was increased to 50 % of ILP during the first two weeks for beginners (BG). During the third and fourth weeks intensity was increased to 60 % of ILP and to 70 % of ILP during the final two weeks. Advanced athletes (AT) performed both exercises at 70 % of ILP during weeks one and two, 80 % during weeks three and four and 90 % of ILP during weeks five and six. After these six weeks both groups were tested again on both exercises. For all pre-tests and post-tests the same testing procedure was used.

Table 3: Test design for the two different training groups

	beginners	advanced athletes
week 1 - 2	familiarization	
week 3	ILP-Test (12-RM)	
week 4 - 5	50 % ILP	70 % ILP
week 6 - 7	60 % ILP	80 % ILP
week 8 - 9	70 % ILP	90 % ILP
week 10	ILP-Retest (12-RM)	

Data analysis

Mean and standard deviation data was presented for all subject characteristics. Percent and frequency curve was calculated. One Sample t-test was used to identify significant differences among test and retest. An alpha level less than or equal to 0.05 was required for statistical significance.

Results

Beginners (BG) realised an average strength increase of 19,36 % for bench presses ($t = 11.47$; $p < 0.05$) and 20,50 % for leg presses ($t = 11.37$; $p < 0.05$) (cf. table 4).

Table 4: Increase in bench press and leg press for BG

	increase bench press (%)	increase leg press (%)
mean	19.36	20.5
SD	4.84	5.1
minimum	13	14
maximum	27	29

Advanced athletes (AT) improved their strength by 13,88 % for both exercises (bench presses: $t = 7.12$; $p < 0.05$; leg presses: $t = 8.88$; $p < 0.05$) (cf. table 5).

Table 5: Increase in bench press and leg press performance for AT

	increase bench press (%)	increase leg press (%)
mean	13.88	13.88
SD	5.51	4.42
minimum	5	7
maximum	20	19

One subject (BG) increased her strength by 29 % for the leg presses. One subject in the AT group increased his strength by 20 % for the bench presses. The lowest increase was found in the BG group where one subject increased his strength by only 13 % for bench presses. In the AT group the lowest increase was an increase by 5 % for bench presses (cf. tables 6 - 9).

Table 6: Test results and training intensity for bench presses for beginners (week 1 to 6; 2 training sessions per week; 3 sets à 12 repetitions) (f = female; m = male)

subject	test 1	week 1 - 2 50 % ILP	week 3 - 4 60 % ILP	week 5 - 6 70 % ILP	test 2
1 (f)	16 kg	8 kg	9.5 kg	11.5 kg	19 kg
2 (m)	39 kg	20 kg	23 kg	27 kg	44 kg
3 (m)	44 kg	22 kg	26 kg	31 kg	55 kg
4 (m)	50 kg	25 kg	30 kg	35 kg	58 kg
5 (f)	24 kg	12 kg	14 kg	17 kg	29 kg
6 (m)	43 kg	21.5 kg	26 kg	30 kg	52 kg
7 (f)	26 kg	13 kg	16 kg	18 kg	33 kg
8 (m)	48 kg	24 kg	29 kg	34 kg	55 kg

Table 7: Test results and training intensity for leg press exercise for the beginners (week 1 to 6; 2 training sessions per week; 3 sets à 12 repetitions) (f = female; m = male)

subject	test 1	week 1 - 2 50 % ILP	week 3 - 4 60 % ILP	week 5 - 6 70 % ILP	test 2
1 (f)	85 kg	42.5 kg	51 kg	60 kg	110 kg
2 (m)	120 kg	60 kg	72 kg	84 kg	142 kg
3 (m)	182 kg	91 kg	109 kg	127 kg	208 kg
4 (m)	158 kg	79 kg	95 kg	110 kg	185 kg
5 (f)	116 kg	58 kg	70 kg	81 kg	140 kg
6 (m)	152 kg	76 kg	91 kg	107 kg	179 kg
7 (f)	110 kg	55 kg	66 kg	77 kg	140 kg
8 (m)	138 kg	69 kg	83 kg	97 kg	166 kg

Table 8: Test results and training intensity for bench press exercise for the advanced athletes (week 1 to 6; 2 training sessions per week; 3 sets à 12 repetitions)

subject	test 1	week 1 - 2 70 % ILP	week 3 - 4 80 % ILP	week 5 - 6 90 % ILP	test 2
1 (m)	40 kg	28 kg	32 kg	36 kg	48 kg
2 (m)	54 kg	38 kg	43 kg	49 kg	62 kg
3 (m)	94 kg	66 kg	75 kg	85 kg	100 kg
4 (m)	61 kg	43 kg	49 kg	55 kg	70 kg
5 (m)	69 kg	48 kg	55 kg	62 kg	80 kg
6 (m)	50 kg	35 kg	40 kg	45 kg	58 kg
7 (m)	61 kg	43 kg	49 kg	55 kg	64 kg
8 (m)	58 kg	40 kg	46 kg	52 kg	69 kg

Table 9: Test results and training intensity for leg press exercise for the advanced athletes (week 1 to 6; 2 training sessions per week; 3 sets à 12 repetitions)

subject	test 1	week 1 - 2 70 % ILP	week 3 - 4 80 % ILP	week 5 - 6 90 % ILP	test 2
1 (m)	147 kg	103 kg	118 kg	132 kg	173 kg
2 (m)	165 kg	115 kg	132 kg	149 kg	185 kg
3 (m)	231 kg	162 kg	185 kg	208 kg	257 kg
4 (m)	150 kg	105 kg	120 kg	135 kg	179 kg
5 (m)	205 kg	144 kg	164 kg	185 kg	226 kg
6 (m)	126 kg	88 kg	101 kg	113 kg	147 kg
7 (m)	173 kg	121 kg	138 kg	156 kg	185 kg
8 (m)	165 kg	115 kg	132 kg	149 kg	193 kg

Discussion

In this study increases in strength and work load were used in order to evaluate the effectiveness of the respective training method applied. However, it soon became obvious that there is no actual guideline that could be applied in order to evaluate the effectiveness of a given training method. This study found average strength increases of close to 20 %. It has been suggested in the literature that increases of 20 % should be achieved during this timescale (cf. Anderson & Kearney, 1982, p. 1ff; Berger, 1962, p. 168ff; Brown & Harrison, 1986, p. 315ff; Rutherford & Jones, 1986, p. 110ff). Judged on practical experience and the literature mentioned above the subjects in this study made considerable progress. However, due to different study designs (testing parameters, the subjects' level of performance etc.) conclusions can hardly be drawn as to whether or not the progress the subjects made in this particular study is above average or not.

One aspect that should be taken into consideration is that training intensity was kept remarkably low during the first weeks of the study (50 % of ILP in the BG group during week one and 60 % during week two) which is congruent with the concept of "moderate strength training" by Buskies (1999; 2001). Further studies are needed to find out whether there are overreaching effects (Schmidtbleicher & Haralambie, 1981) and whether these implications might also be relevant for very advanced or even elite athletes. In addition to that, these results would also have to be compared to training programs that include HITM (Gießing, 2004).

Conclusion

In contrast to the usual recommendations (Bührle, 1985; Zatsiorsky, 1996) the ILP method may be used by athletes of all levels of performance. By adjusting training parameters accordingly it is made sure that there is not too much strain on the organism and therefore the risk of injury is kept to a minimum. As the athletes' performances improve, training parameters are adjusted accordingly.

Training intensity and work load for all exercises are always calculated based on initial submaximal ILP tests instead of 1-RM tests which is also a much safer procedure especially for beginners (Braith, Graves, Leggett, & Pollock,

1993). Cardiovascular and metabolic stress is expected to be in an acceptable range for fitness- and recreational athletes. Terminating sets before the PMF has been reached further reduces cardiovascular stress as well as stress on the joints (Buskies, 1999; Stone, Chandler, Conley, Kramer, & Stone, 1996). The training parameters applied in ILP training make it easier to begin and continue a training program since it takes motivational factors into consideration. According to Prochaska, DiClemente and Norcross (1994) this is of great importance during the first six months after, newly beginning a training program. Another factor that has a positive effect on motivation is that athletes have to write down their training results and therefore receive valuable feedback concerning their improvements. In order to collect more empirical data on the value of the ILP method, further research is needed that studies the results produced by this method using a greater number of subjects and studying the effects of the ILP method over a longer timescale that includes a whole macrocycle during which athletes alternate putting the emphasis on strength, hypertrophy and muscle strength endurance.

References

Anderson, T., & Kearney, J. T. (1982). Effects of three resistance training programs on muscular strength and absolute and relative endurance. *Research Quarterly for Exercise and Sport, 53*(1), 1-7.

Berger, R. A. (1962). Effect of varied weight training programs on strength. *The Research Quarterly, 33*(2), 168-181.

Borg, G. (2004). Anstrengungsempfinden und körperliche Aktivität [Perceived exertion and physical activity]. *Deutsches Ärzteblatt, 101*(15), A1016-A1021.

Braith, R. W., Graves, J. E., Leggett, S. H., & Pollock, M. L. (1993). Effect of training on the relationship between maximal and submaximal strength. *Medicine & Science in Sports & Exercise, 25*(1), 132-138.

Brown, R. D., & Harrison, J. M. (1986). The effects of a strength training program on the strength and self concept of two female age groups. *Research Quarterly for Exercise and Sport, 57*(4), 315-320.

Bührle, M. (1985). *Grundlagen des Maximal- und Schnellkrafttrainings [Fundamentals of maximum strength and power training]*. Schorndorf: Hofmann.

Buskies, W. (1999). Sanftes Krafttraining nach dem subjektiven Belastungsempfinden versus Training bis zur muskulären Ausbelastung [Moderate strength training regulated by RPE versus training until muscle exhaustion]. *Deutsche Zeitschrift für Sportmedizin, 50*(10), 316-320.

Buskies, W. (2001). Zur Bedeutung des sanften Krafttrainings nach dem subjektiven Belastungsempfinden [The importance of moderate strength training regulated by RPE]. *Sportwissenschaft, 31*(1), 45-60.

Buskies, W., & Boeckh-Behrens, W.-U. (1999). Probleme bei der Steuerung der Trainingsintensität im Krafttraining auf der Basis von Maximalkrafttests [Problems concerning the management of training intensity in strength training]. *Leistungssport, 29*(3), 4-8.

De Lorme, T. L. (1945). Restoration of muscle power by heavy-resistance exercises. *Journal of Bone and Joint Surgery, 27*(4), 645-667.

Denner, A. (1998). *Analyse und Training der wirbelsäulenstabilisierenden Muskulatur [Analysis and training of spine stabilising muscles]*. Berlin, Heidelberg: Springer.

Eifler, C. (2000). *Krafttraining nach der "Individuellen-Leistungsbild-Methode" - eine empirische Überprüfung der Trainingseffekte bei Anfängern und Fortgeschrittenen [Strength training according to the "Individual Lifting Performance Method" - an empirical review of training effects on beginners and advanced subjects]*. Unpublished diplomathesis, Universität des Saarlandes, Saarbrücken.

Fleck, S. J. (2002). Periodization of training. In W. J. Kraemer & K. Häkkinen (Eds.), *Handbook of sports medicine and science. Strength training for sport* (pp. 55-68). Oxford: Blackwell Science Ltd.

Fleck, S. J., & Kraemer, W. J. (2004). *Designing resistance training programs* (3rd ed.). Champaign, IL: Human Kinetics.

Fröhlich, M. (2003). *Kraftausdauertraining. Eine empirische Studie zur Methodik [Strength endurance training. An empirical study]*. Göttingen: Cuvillier.

Fröhlich, M., Klein, M., Emrich, E., & Schmidtbleicher, D. (2001). Arbeit als Bruttokriterium der Belastung im Kraftausdauertraining [Work as gross criterium of the work load in strength endurance training]. *Leistungssport, 31*(2), 24-28.

Fukunaga, T. (1976). Die absolute Muskelkraft und das Muskeltraining [Absolute strength and muscle training]. *Sportarzt und Sportmedizin, 11*, 255-262.

Gießing, J. (2004). *1 Satz Training - Ein wissenschaftlich fundiertes Konzept für schnellstmöglichen Muskelaufbau im Bodybuilding [Single-set training. A concept for rapid muscle gains based on scientific findings]* (1st ed.). Arnsberg: Novagenics.

Hoeger, W. W. K., Barette, S. L., Hale, D. F., & Hopkins, D. R. (1987). Relationship between repetitions and selected percentages of one repetition maximum. *Journal of Applied Sports Science Research, 1*(1), 11-13.

Hoeger, W. W. K., Hopkins, D. R., Barette, S. L., & Hale, D. F. (1990). Relationship between repetitions and selected percentages of one repetition maximum: A comparison between untrained and trained males and females. *Journal of Applied Sport Science Research, 4*(2), 47-54.

Kempf, H.-D., & Strack, A. (2001). *Der Hantel Krafttrainer [The barbell strength trainer]*. Reinbek: Rowohlt.

Komi, P. V. (1986). Training of muscle strength and power: Interaction of neuromotoric, hypertropic, and mechanical factors. *International Journal of Sports Medicine, 7*(1), S10-15.

Kraemer, W. J., & Fry, A. C. (1995). Strength testing: Development and evaluation of methodology. In P. J. Maud & C. Foster (Eds.), *Physiological assessment of human submaximal Intensität* (pp. 115-138). Champaign IL: Human Kinetics.

MacDougall, J. D., Elder, G. C., Sale, D. G., Moroz, J. R., & Sutton, J. R. (1980). Effects of strength training and immobilization on human muscle fibres. *European Journal of Applied Physiolgy and Occupational Physiolgy, 43*(1), 25-34.

Marschall, F., & Fröhlich, M. (1999). Überprüfung des Zusammenhangs von Maximalkraft und maximaler Wiederholungszahl bei deduzierten submaximalen Intensitäten [Testing the correlation between maximal strength and repetition maximum for deduced lower levels of intensity]. *Deutsche Zeitschrift für Sportmedizin, 50*(10), 311-315.

Pette, D. (1999). Das adaptative Potential des Skelettmuskels [The adaptative potential of skeletal muscle]. *Deutsche Zeitschrift für Sportmedizin, 50*(9), 262-271.

Prochaska, O. M., DiClemente, C. C., & Norcross, J. C. (1994). *Changing for goog. A revolutionary six-stage-program for overcoming bad habits and moving your life positively forward.* New York: Harper Collind.

Rutherford, O. M., & Jones, D. A. (1986). The role of learning and coordination in strength training. *European Journal of Applied Physiology, 55*, 100-105.

Schlumberger, A., & Schmidtbleicher, D. (1999). Einsatz-Training als trainingsmethodische Alternative - Möglichkeiten und Grenzen [Single-set training as methodical alternative - potentials and limits]. *Leistungssport, 29*(3), 9-11.

Schmidtbleicher, D., & Haralambie, G. (1981). Changes in contractile properties of muscle after strength training in man. *European Journal of Applied Physiology, 46*, 211-219.

Stone, M. H., Chandler, T. J., Conley, M. S., Kramer, J. B., & Stone, M. E. (1996). Training to muscular failure: Is it necessary? *Strength and Conditioning, 18*(3), 44-48.

Strack, A. (1998a). Krafttrainingsmethoden-Dschungel. Betriebswirtschaftlich oder trainingswissenschaftlich orientierte Krafttrainingsmethodik im Fitness-Studio? [Jungle of strength training methods. Business or sport scientific orientated strength training methods in fitness clubs? *Trainer, 4*, 16-31.

Strack, A. (1998b). Methodik des modernen Krafttraining im Fitness- und Gesundheitssport [Methods of modern strength training in fitness and health sports]. *Trainer, 3*, 11-14.

Strack, A. (1999). Individuelle Leistungsmethode im wissenschaftlichen Test [Scientific examination of the Individual Lifting Performance Method]. *Trainer*, 41-44.

Strack, A. (2000). *Gesundheits- und fitnessorientiertes Krafttraining nach Individuellen-Leistungsbild-Methode [Health and fitness orientated strength training accordingly to the Individual Lifting Performance Method].* Trier: Congress für Sporttherapie, Physiotherapie und Fitness 14-16.4.2000.

Zatsiorsky, V. M. (1996). *Krafttraining - Wissenschaft und Praxis [Science and practice of strength training].* Aachen: Meyer & Meyer.

MARKUS KLEIN, MICHAEL FRÖHLICH & JÜRGEN GIEßING

A theoretical concept for quantifying the effectiveness of muscle endurance training

Keywords: muscle endurance training, prediction, work load, repetition, testing

Introduction

For most athletes strength and power are of outstanding importance for their performance (Martin, Carl, & Lehnertz, 1993, p. 100), especially in competitive sports in which an athlete's performance can be measured exactly such as track and field, swimming, and weightlifting. However, strength and power are also important in sports such as gymnastics where the athletes have to perform certain movements which require a certain amount of strength and power (Sands, McNeal, Jenni, & Delong, 2000). In addition to this, more and more attention is being paid to developing strength and muscle mass for injury prevention, rehabilitation and general well-being (Zimmermann, 2000). This development is generally regarded as a reaction to the progressive decline of physical activity which usually accompanies the ageing process. Another factor that contributes to this is the technological progress because of which there is hardly any necessity for physical activity in daily living (Buskies, 1999; Klein, 2000).

Especially the loss of strength during ageing is attributed to a reduced amount of physical activity (Kolb, 1999). For elderly people in particular, declining strength levels as a result of less physical activity make many activities of daily living even harder which in turn leads to a further decline in strength, creating a vicious circle that results in a progressive decline of strength. This is exactly why a well-planned muscle training program can help elderly people cope with the necessities of daily living. Such a program should be aimed at improving muscle endurance (Zimmermann, 2000) and should be intense enough to induce a positive kind of adaptation without putting an undesired amount of stress on the neural, muscosceletal and cardiovascular system (Urhausen, Schwarz, Stefan, Gabriel, & Kindermann, 2000).

In addition to these aspects, muscle endurance training can be used as the foundation for other training methods such as muscle hypertrophy training or

training for improving intramuscular and intermuscular coordination (Boeckh-Behrens & Buskies, 1998, p. 42).
However, both scientific and empirical evidence concerning muscle endurance training are inconsistent and sometimes even contradictory (Fröhlich, Klein, Emrich, & Schmidtbleicher, 2001) which makes designing muscle endurance programs difficult since different training designs will inevitably result in different kinds of adaptation. This is why it is difficult to compare different training designs and their results. Radlinger, Bachmann, Homburg, Leuenberger and Thaddey (1998) refer to Hollmann and Hettinger (1990) and distinguish between subjective, semi-objective, and objective testing procedures. Taking all these aspects into consideration, it must be stated that there are several testing procedures which are also suitable for testing muscle endurance.

Muscle strength endurance

A review of the literature that deals with muscle endurance training shows a considerable variety of definitions for muscle endurance (Fröhlich et al., 2001). Carl, Starischka and Stork (1989, p. 3) criticise that there is a tremendous lack of findings concerning developing muscle endurance. Results of empirical studies are inconsistent concerning training design and methods for improving muscle endurance in a number of studies (Harre, 1986; Hollmann & Hettinger, 1990; Martin et al., 1993; Nicolaus, 1993; Pampus, Lehnertz, & Martin, 1989; Schmidtbleicher, 1987; Schnabel, Harre, & Borde, 1997; Weineck, 1994).
The German term for "muscle endurance" is "Kraftausdauer" which translates into "muscle strength endurance" and puts an emphasis on the strength aspect. In his famous book "Trainingslehre" Harre (1986) defines muscle strength endurance as the ability to resist fatigue in strength training for a longer duration. Harre (1986) characterises muscle strength endurance as a combination of strength and endurance. He recommends a high training volume and resistances which are greater than those used in competition. Harre also prefers the design suggested by Scholich (1974) that consists of a circle training using weights of 40 to 60 % of 1-RM which can be lifted 25 to 50 times per set. Ehlenz, Grosser and Zimmermann (1998) largely agree with this, however, they distinguish between what they call maximum strength endurance that should be trained with resistances of at least 75 % of 1-RM, submaximal strength endurance that should be trained with 75 to 50 % of 1-RM and aerobic muscle endurance that should be trained with 50 to 30 % of 1-RM.

Neither Harre (1986) nor Ehlenz et al. (1998) do provide any information concerning time under tension (TUT). Most of the recent definitions of muscle strength endurance training refer to Schmidtbleicher (1987) and Schmidtbleicher (1989) who defines muscle strength endurance as the ability of the neuromuscular system to tolerate as large a sum of impulses as possible over a certain amount of time (no more than two minutes when maximum effort is applied with a resistance of at least 30 % of 1-RM. Schmidtbleicher further points out that the reduction of the impulses produced should be as low as possible. Recent publications like the one by Güllich and Schmidtbleicher (1999) emphasise that muscle strength endurance consists of two components. One component being the extent of any single strength impulse and the other one being the ability of keeping the reduction in the sum of all single impulses as low as possible. The extent of a single impulse depends to a great extend on an individual´s strength, whereas the ability of keeping the reduction in the sum of all single impulses low is directly related to the tolerance and clearance of lactic acid as well as to neural factors. The following table shows the authors´ recommendations concerning configurations for muscle strength endurance training.

Table 1: Configurations for muscle strength endurance training (Güllich & Schmidtbleicher, 1999, p. 232)

muscle strength endurance method	
intensity (% of 1-RM)	50 to 60 %
repetitions per set	20 to 40
sets per workout (per muscle group)	6 to 8
rest between sets	0.5 to 1 min
velocity of the movement	controlled

Fröhlich et al. (2001) emphasise the importance of the time under tension (TUT) and point out that TUT is such an important factor that it has to be considered when choosing the appropriate resistance for a certain exercise. For a muscle strength endurance training program a TUT of 45 to 60 seconds should be chosen. In same cases a longer TUT seems to make sense, e. g. in the muscle strength endurance training of competitive rowers who sometimes apply a TUT of up to two minutes. The velocity of each repetition should be the same. Repetitions between 25 and 30 are usually recommended. For each set a resistance should be chosen that allows for the desired number of repetitions and remains within the TUT mentioned above.

Problems in testing muscle strength endurance

In practical training in general as well as in determining muscle strength endurance in particular, subjective, semi-subjective and objective testing procedures are applied (Hollmann & Hettinger, 1990). In addition to this, so-called clinical-functional strength tests are applied which are supposed to provide information about the strength and power of the large muscle groups. However practical these clinical-functional tests may be, some problems arise when the theoretical background of testing is taken into consideration (Radlinger et al., 1998). State-of-the-art electronical testing devices as well as some mechanical testing devices produce results that are highly reliable in measuring all kinds of strength, however, operating these machines is often difficult and expensive. The same can be said about testing procedures that take isometrical tests during a given time-span which is even more difficult to realise because of the technical equipment needed (Ballreich & Baumann, 1996). Because of all these difficulties there is the need for testing procedures that are both inexpensive and not to difficult to realise in a practical training environment. Therefore the following theoretical concept for quantifying the efficiency of muscle strength endurance training was developed.

Components of muscle strength endurance

One way of determining improvements in muscle strength endurance is realising more repetitions with the same resistance than in previous workouts. There is also an improvement in muscle strength endurance if the same number of repetitions can be realised after the resistance for that exercise had been increased. This means that improvements in muscle strength endurance become obvious either by an increase in repetition maximums with an unchanged resistance which focuses on the endurance aspect of muscle strength endurance or by using heavier resistances for the same number of repetitions which focuses more on the strength aspect.
The number of repetitions can be used in order to calculate the sum of the range of motion over which of the resistance is moved in all sets and to calculate the total work load (*range of motion x repetitions x resistance*). Figure 1 shows the relationship between work load [N], repetitions [reps] and the range

of motion over which the weight was moved [m]. These parameters clearly indicate the status quo of the training session.

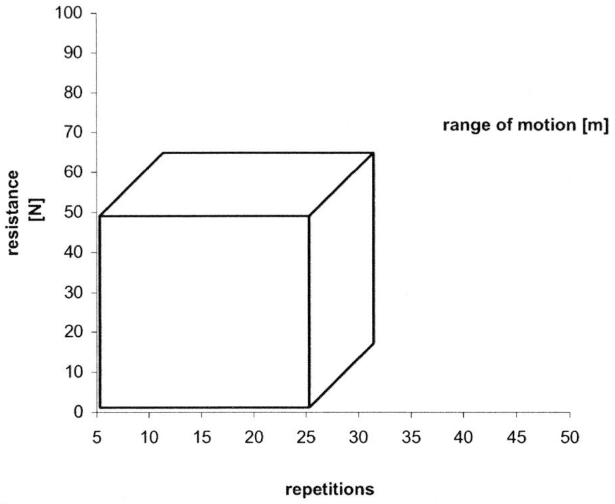

Figure 1: Relationship between work load [N], repetitions [reps] and the range of motion over which the weight was moved [m]

By looking at the external criteria "physical work" [Nm] training sessions can be analysed which offers opportunities to compare different training methods, their effectiveness can be analysed and the progress a trainee makes on a certain training program can be evaluated.

Quantifying the effectiveness of muscle strength endurance training

Based on the theoretical background explained above which differentiates between an emphasis on the endurance aspect and a strength aspect of muscle strength endurance training, two different approaches for quantifying progress in muscle strength endurance. Both procedures require a pre-test at the beginning of each training period. After conclusion of the training period a post-test that tests the number of repetitions with the same resistance used in the pre-test will show the improvement that has been made. These changes in the number of repetitions will then demonstrate the effectiveness of the program in terms of evaluating the endurance aspect, whereas testing the maximum resistance that can be lifted as many times as the weight in the pre-test was lifted would be used in order to test the strength aspect of a given muscle strength endurance training program as shown in figure 2.

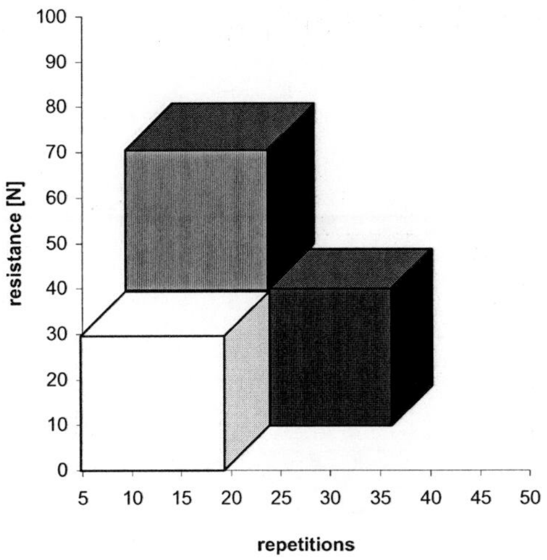

Figure 2: Quantifying the effectiveness of muscle strength endurance training programs through an increase of repetitions with the same resistance or the difference in resistance that can be lifted for the same number of repetitions

The following sample calculation shows possible training effects of a muscle strength endurance training program (cf. Fröhlich, 2003, p. 202):

Pre-test: Determining maximum resistance y_1 lifted for a maximum of x_1 repetitions over a certain range of motion s_1

<u>sample calculation</u>:

x_1 = 25 repetitions

s_1 = 0.4 meters (bench presses)

y_1 = 500 N (maximum resistance for 25 repetitions)

$f_{\text{(pre-test)}} = x_1 \times s_1 \times y_1$

$f_{\text{(pre-test)}} = 25 \times 0.4 \times 500$ [reps × m × N]

$f_{\text{(pre-test)}} = 5000$ [Nm]

This sample calculation is based on an example in which 500 [N] could be bench pressed 25 times over a range of motion of 0.4 meters (from chest to full extension of both arms) and thereby producing 5000 [Nm].

If the trainee trained for six weeks bench pressing three times a week using a weight that he can lift 30 times for three sets, the effectiveness of this training program could then be tested in two different ways:

Post-test 1: Determining the maximum resistance y_2 for x_1 and s_1

sample calculation 1: $f_{(post\text{-}test)} = x_1 \times s_1 \times y_2$

$f_{(post\text{-}test)} = 25 \times 0.4 \times 600$

$f_{(post\text{-}test)} = 6000$ Nm

E (effectiveness 1) = $x_1 \times (y_2 - y_1) \times s_1 = 1000$ Nm (focussing on strength aspect)

Post-test 2: Determining the maximum number of repetitions x_2 with y_1 and s_1

sample calculation 2: $f_{(post\text{-}test)} = x_2 \times s_1 \times y_1$

$f_{(post\text{-}test)} = 40 \times 0.4 \times 500$

$f_{(post\text{-}test)} = 8000$ Nm

E (effectiveness 2) = $y_1 \times (x_2 - x_1) \times s_1 = 3000$ Nm (focussing on endurance aspect)

Whereas sample calculation 1 shows an increase of maximum resistance y_2 and focuses more on the strength aspect of muscle strength endurance training, the setting of sample calculation 2 is obviously more focused on the endurance aspect. It would be interesting to see if actual training programs would produce similar results as the ones shown in the sample calculation. Another question is if both aspects can be targeted individually. These questions can only be answered by applying this theoretical concept on actual training programs and comparing the results to the ones of these calculations.

References

Ballreich, R., & Baumann, W. (1996). *Grundlagen der Biomechanik des Sports [Fundamentals of biomechanics in sports]*. Stuttgart: Enke.

Boeckh-Behrens, W.-U., & Buskies, W. (1998). *Gesundheitsorientiertes Fitnesstraining [Health-orientate fitness strength training]* (1st ed.). Lüneburg: Wehdemeier & Pusch.

Buskies, W. (1999). *Sanftes Krafttraining. Unter besonderer Berücksichtigung des subjektiven Belastungsempfindens [Moderate strength training. Under special consideration of the rate of perceived exertion]*. Köln: Sport und Buch Strauß.

Carl, K., Starischka, S., & Stork, H.-M. (1989). *Kraftausdauertraining [Strength endurance training]*. Köln: Sport und Buch Strauß.

Ehlenz, H., Grosser, M., & Zimmermann, E. (1998). *Krafttraining. Grundlagen, Methoden, Übungen, Leistungssteuerung, Trainingsprogramme [Strength training. Basics, methods, exercises, performance management, training programs]* (6th ed.). München: BLV Sportwissen.

Fröhlich, M. (2003). *Kraftausdauertraining. Eine empirische Studie zur Methodik [Strength endurance training. An empirical study]*. Göttingen: Cuvillier.

Fröhlich, M., Klein, M., Emrich, E., & Schmidtbleicher, D. (2001). Arbeit als Bruttokriterium der Belastung im Kraftausdauertraining [Work as gross criterium of the work load in strength endurance training]. *Leistungssport, 31*(2), 24-28.

Güllich, A., & Schmidtbleicher, D. (1999). Struktur der Kraftfähigkeiten und ihrer Trainingsmethoden [Structure of motor strength and the training methods]. *Deutsche Zeitschrift für Sportmedizin, 50*(7+8), 223-234.

Harre, D. (1986). *Trainingslehre: Einführung in die Theorie und Methodik des sportlichen Trainings [Conditioning science. Introduction in theory and methods of training]* (10th ed.). Berlin: Sportverlag.

Hollmann, W., & Hettinger, T. (1990). *Sportmedizin - Arbeits und Trainingsgrundlagen [Sports medicine - labour and training fundamentals]* (3rd ed.). Stuttgart, New York: Schattauer.

Klein, M. (2000). *Zum Einfluss maximaler und submaximaler Trainingsbelastungen auf die Veränderung der Relativkraft und die Wiederholungsanzahl bei submaximalen Lasten [Influence of maximal and submaximal training load on changes in relative strength and number of repetitions with submaximal loads]*. Unpublished diplomathesis, Universität des Saarlandes, Saarbrücken.

Kolb, M. (1999). *Bewegtes Altern - Grundlagen und Perspektiven einer Sportgeragogik [Active aging - fundamentals and perspectives in sports geragogic*. Schorndorf: Hofmann.

Martin, D., Carl, K., & Lehnertz, K. (1993). *Handbuch Trainingslehre [Handbook training science]* (2nd. ed.). Schorndorf: Hofmann.

Nicolaus, J. (1993). Kenngrößen der Kraftausdauer - Qualifizierung und Quantifizierung anhand des Zweiphasen-Tests [Parameters of strength endurance - qualification and quantification by a two phases test]. In D. Martin & S. Weigelt (Eds.), *Trainingswissenschaft - Selbstverständnis und Forschungsansätze [Training sciences - self-conception and research approaches]* (pp. 130-135). St. Augustin: Academia.

Pampus, B., Lehnertz, K., & Martin, D. (1989). Die Wirkung unterschiedlicher Belastungsintensitäten auf die Entwicklung von Maximalkraft und Kraftausdauer [The influence of different intensities on maximum strength and strength endurance development]. *Leistungssport, 19*(4), 5-10.

Radlinger, L., Bachmann, W., Homburg, J., Leuenberger, U., & Thaddey, G. (1998). *Rehabilitatives Krafttraining [Rehabilitative strength training]*. Stuttgart, New York: Thieme Verlag.

Sands, W. A., McNeal, J. R., Jenni, M., & Delong, T. H. (2000). Should female gymnasts lift weights? *Sportscience, 4*(3), sportsci.org/jour/0003/was.html.

Schmidtbleicher, D. (1987). Motorische Beanspruchungsform Kraft [The structure of motor strength]. *Deutsche Zeitschrift für Sportmedizin, 38*(9), 356-377.

Schmidtbleicher, D. (1989). Zum Problem der Definition des Begriffs Kraftausdauer [Problems with the definition of strength endurance training]. In K. Carl, S. Starischka & H.-M. Storck (Eds.), *Kraftausdauertraining [Strength endurance training]* (pp. 10-30). Köln: Sport und Buch Strauß.

Schnabel, G., Harre, D., & Borde, A. (1997). *Trainingswissenschaft [Conditioning science].* Berlin: Sportverlag.

Scholich, M. (1974). *Kreistraining [Circle training].* Frankfurt am Main: Bartels & Wernitz.

Urhausen, A., Schwarz, M., Stefan, S., Gabriel, H., & Kindermann, W. (2000). Kardiovaskuläre und metabolische Beanspruchung durch einen Kraftausdauer-Zirkel in der ambulanten Herztherapie [Cardiovascular and metabolic strain during a strength-endurance circle training in out-patient cardiac rehabilitation]. *Deutsche Zeitschrift für Sportmedizin, 51*(4), 130-136.

Weineck, J. (1994). *Optimales Training [Optimal training]* (8th ed.). Balingen: PERIMED-spitta.

Zimmermann, K. (2000). *Gesundheitsorientiertes Muskelkrafttraining [Health-orientated strength training].* Schorndorf: Hofmann.

STEPHEN GLASS & DOUGLAS STANTON

Self selected resistance training intensity in novice weight lifters

Keywords: exercise prescription, strength training, % 1-RM, lifting intensity, load

Introduction

Effective resistance training programs involve a combination of adequate overload stimulus, and repetitive volume. Research has indicated that a load of 60 - 75 percent of an individual's 1-repetition-maximum (1-RM) is required to induce strength gain and muscle hypertrophy (ACSM, 2000; Fleck & Kraemer, 1997). Loads under 60 % are generally ineffective for producing strength gains. Common exercise prescription methodology in resistance training involves the use of an initial 1-RM or perhaps 6-RM test to establish maximal strength for a given lift. Training intensity is then based upon a percentage of maximum. In the health and fitness setting, individuals are often not able to complete 1-RM testing, either due to a lack of personnel to test clients, a lack of time or risks associated with untrained individuals performing 1-RM testing. As a result, many individuals are provided an orientation as to the proper form and order of exercises, and then self select training load to begin their resistance training program. It is unclear whether individuals are able to choose an appropriate resistance training load without initial 1-RM or 6-RM testing.

Research has examined effectiveness of intensity self-selection in aerobic exercise. Studies have generally asked individuals to choose an intensity that they feel will provide a "good cardiovascular stimulus" (Dishman, Farquhar, & Cureton, 1994; Glass & Chvala, 2001; Kravitz, Robergs, Heyward, Wagner, & Powers, 1997; Melanson, Freedson, Webb, Jungbluth, & Kozlowski, 1996; Spelman, Pate, Macera, & Ward, 1993) without any prior pacing or testing to provide intensity anchors. Subjects then are allowed a time to choose a pace they feel is appropriate, and then exercise for at least 20 minutes. Using this methodology Dishman et al. (1994) found that both high and low fit individuals selected exercise intensities that were close to 60 % VO_{2peak}.

Subsequently, Glass and Chvala (2001) found that when mode of exercise was manipulated, subjects again chose approximately 55 - 60 % VO_{2peak} for treadmill, cycling and stair-stepping exercise. These intensities are within the low range of effective conditioning intensity as suggested by the American College of Sports Medicine (2000). Perception of effort and self-regulation of exercise intensity during resistance training is a relatively new area of research. A number of studies have examined perceptual responses to assigned percentages of 1-RM (estimation studies), and have demonstrated a linear relationship between work intensity and perception of effort (Gearhart et al., 2002; Lagally et al., 2002; O´Conner, Poudevigne, & Pasley, 2002; Pincivero, Coelho, & Erikson, 2000). Lagally et al. (2002) examined the RPE, blood lactate and electromyographic responses to bicep curl exercise at 30 %, 60 % and 90 % 1-RM in women. They found that both RPE overall as well as RPE for the active muscle increased significantly across load intensities, with the active muscle displaying significantly higher RPE values than the overall scores. Similarly, Gearhart et al. (2001) found that active muscle RPE was significantly greater during a high intensity protocol (90 % 1-RM) than low intensity (30 % 1-RM) when total work was held constant. In the instances of these RPE estimation studies, all training was preceded by some type of strength assessment, which serves to provide load perception anchors for the individuals lifting.

Data regarding self-selected weight lifting intensities are relatively scarce, with most studies related to effects on anxiety. Studies have shown that weight training at light loads (50 % 1-RM) can positively influence state anxiety (Bartholomew & Linder, 1998; Focht, 2002; Focht & Koltyn, 2000), while heavy loads actually increase anxiety. This may cause individuals to choose lighter training loads. Focht (2002) examined state anxiety among novice female weight lifters following prescribed (75 % 1-RM) and self selected exercise intensity (56 % 1-RM). Results showed a decline in state anxiety only following the self selected lifting intensity. This is consistent among other research that has prescribed light weight lifting intensities (40 - 60 % 1-RM) (Bartholomew & Linder, 1998; Focht & Koltyn, 2000).

Since subjects in previous studies were first assessed for 1-RM, thus providing intensity anchors, it is not known whether individuals self select light training loads without initial perceptual information. Glass and Holcomb (1997) found that individuals not provided initial pacing or testing chose work intensities far above expected values for their assigned RPE. For individuals who are not provided 1-RM testing at the onset of a program, but are instead instructed to choose a weight that feels “heavy enough to cause an increase in strength”, it is not known whether they will perceptually choose an intensity that is sufficient to induce hypertrophy and strength gain. Based on previous research it is hypothesized that unlike aerobic endurance training, self-selection of weight lifting intensity will not be intense enough to meet general guidelines for strength gain, and thus prove ineffective as a means of exercise programming. Thus the purpose of this study was to determine the intensity of self selected weight lifting exercise in untrained men and women.

Methods

Subjects

Thirteen men (age = 19.54 ± 1.85 y) and 17 women (18.71 ± 1.00 y) were recruited for the study. Subjects provided signed consent in accordance with the Institutional Review Board and were individuals who had not performed any resistance training for the past 6 months. The study was conducted in accordance with the institutional policy for research with human subjects. The group was selected on a volunteer basis through personal contact from a college-age population. All of the subjects were apparently healthy based upon health questionnaire data, and provided written consent to complete the study. All subjects completed an initial orientation day, where resting characteristics were measured and subjects were provided a weight training orientation. Subjects were set properly for the variable resistance exercises (Badger Magnum Selecterized Equipment) and instructed as to the proper form. Cadence was standardized ("controlled pace" approx. 2 s up, 2 s down) for lifting. Subjects then reported back within 48 h for the first of two weight training days. Following the two training days, subjects' 1-RM were assessed for each lift.

Subject characteristics

Height and weight of subjects (men = 177.8 ± 6.17 cm, 79.3 ± 9.13 kg; women = 164.74 ± 5.89 cm, 61.55 ± 10.34 kg) were measured using a Stadiometer (nearest cm) and a Health-o-meter scale (nearest 0.01 kg) respectively. Men were significantly heavier and taller than women ($p < 0.05$). Skinfold body density was determined (Lange calipers) using the three site Jackson-Pollock equations (Pollock, Schmidt, & Jackson, 1980). Body fat was calculated using the Siri equation (Siri, 1961). Women (23.44 ± 4.74 %) had significantly higher body fat percentages than men (14.27 ± 6.76 %) ($p < 0.05$). Resting systolic and diastolic blood pressure was measured with the subject seated using a standard stethoscope and sphygmomanometer. Men had significantly higher systolic blood pressure (121.31 ± 10.27 mmHg) than women (108.41 ± 10.81 mmHg), with no differences in diastolic pressure (men = 71.85 ± 7.59 mmHg; women = 71.65 ± 8.49 mmHg). Resting heart rate (men = 68.31 ± 13.01 $b \cdot min^{-1}$, women = 76.00 ± 11.49 $b \cdot min^{-1}$) was measured by manual palpation of the radial artery.

Weight training trials

Subjects were provided an orientation regarding Borg's 6 - 20 RPE scale (Borg, 1970). They were instructed to provide an overall rating of their degree of effort during the weight lifting exercise. Then each subject asked to "choose a load that you feel will be sufficient to improve your muscular strength". They were allowed to perform as many repetitions as they wished, and were not given specific instructions to lift to fatigue. Each subject was given as much time as they required in order to select the desired load, however most identified the load within 2 - 3 minutes. Subjects completed 2 sets, with 2 minutes rest between each set. The exercises were performed in the following order:

a) Seated Bench Press,
b) Leg Extension,
c) Seated Back Row,
d) Military Press,
e) Biceps Curl.

Subjects were blinded to the actual weight they lifted, since the researchers placed tape over the markings on the equipment. Forty eight to 72 hours after completing the first weight training session, subjects reported back to the weight room and repeated the same exercise, where they were to again choose their intensity. They were not told what they had chosen the previous trial. All subjects then completed a 1-RM test for each lift within 48 h after the last weight training session.

Data analysis

Load for each lift was recorded, as well as the number of repetitions. Ratings of Perceived Exertion (RPE) was assessed during the second set of exercise for each lift. Following 1-RM testing, the % 1-RM lifted was calculated for each exercise. Data were averaged across sets and the two days of weight lifting (% 1-RM, repetitions, RPE). Data were then compared between gender using independent means t-tests. Significance was set at $p < 0.05$.

Results

Subject characteristics are shown in table 1. Men were significantly taller and heavier than women. Both groups average body fat fell within the desirable range for their gender. Men also displayed a significantly higher systolic blood pressure than women. One repetition max data are shown in table 2. Men showed significantly greater 1-RMs for each lift compared to women. Mean strength to body weight ratios for the bench press 1-RM (men = 1.13; women = 0.61) indicate average strength for the group tested (Heyward, 2002).

*Table 1: One repetition max data (mean ± SD; data expressed in pounds. * = $p < 0.05$)*

lift (muscle group)	men	women
bench (chest)	196.15 ± 39.98	83.09 ± 19.23 *
extension (leg)	198.08 ± 33.01	122.79 ± 26.60 *
pulldown (back)	155.77 ± 19.51	89.71 ± 15.46 *
military press (shoulder)	200.96 ± 36.61	98.53 ± 17.05 *
curl (bicep)	125.38 ± 26.65	54.12 ± 14.60 *

Figure 1 shows the self-selected weight lifting intensity (% 1-RM) chosen by the men and women. Both groups selected intensities that were below 60 % 1-RM for every lift, with no statistical differences between genders.

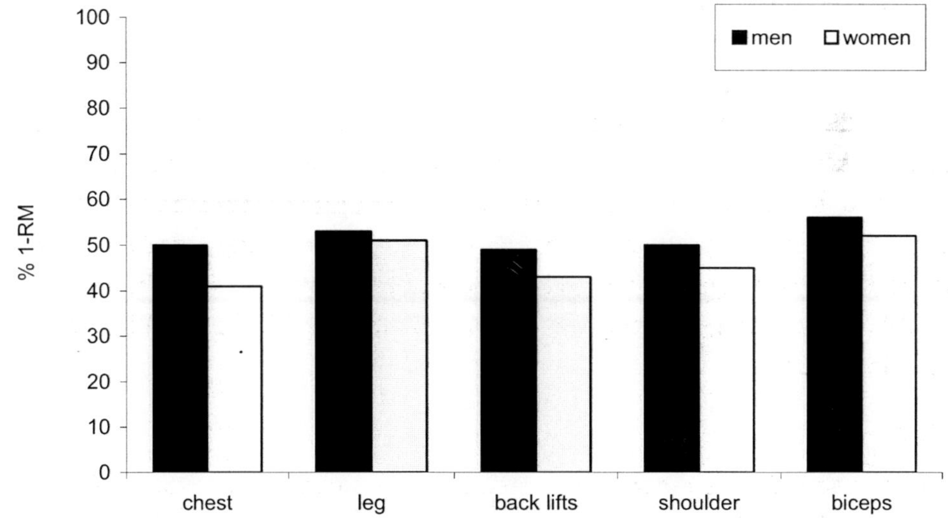

Figure 1: The self-selected weight lifting intensity (% 1-RM) chosen by the men and women

Figure 2 shows the self-selected number of repetitions at the self-selected load. No significant differences were noted between genders, however subjects did not appear to exercise to failure. Instead subjects terminated their exercise between approximately 10 - 25 repetitions, with the fewest repetitions being performed for the shoulder (men = 11.89 ± 2.4; women 12.18 ± 3.6) and biceps (men = 10.62 ± 2.42; women = 9.05 ± 2.91).

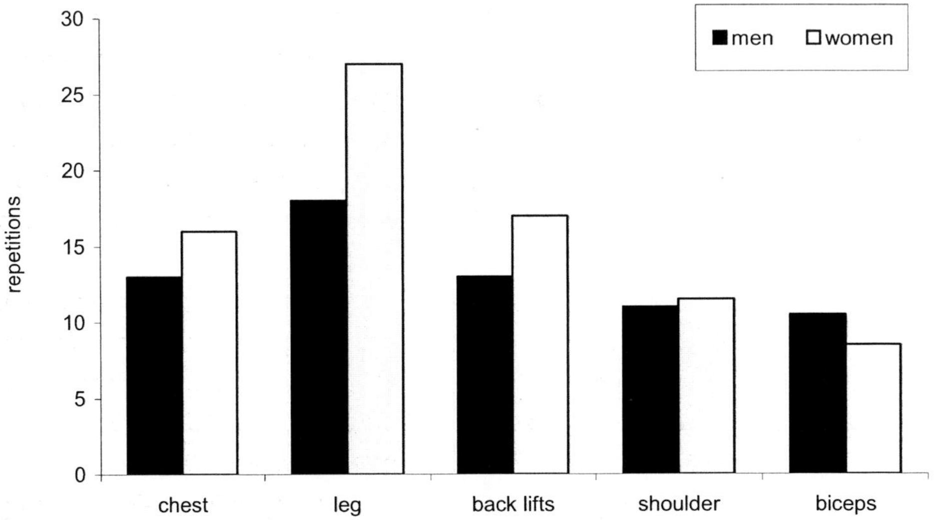

Figure 2: The self-selected number of repetitions at the self-selected load

Table 2 shows the combined results (men and women) for the percent 1-RM lifted and the number of repetitions. It is clear from the results that the subjects chose weights that were too light to overload the muscle, and also did not lift until fatigue. There were no significant differences in RPE between men and women, with both indicating approximately a 13 (somewhat hard) for each lift.

Table 2: Lifting intensity and repetitions completed (mean ± SD)

lift (muscle group)	% 1-RM	repetitions
bench (chest)	45.40 ± 11.14	14.10 ± 6.00
extension (leg)	54.93 ± 13.88	23.30 ± 21.30
pulldown (back)	47.54 ± 0.90	14.47 ± 7.66
military press (shoulder)	48.40 ± 0.92	11.47 ± 2.66
curl (bicep)	42.35 ± 0.50	9.50 ± 2.00

Discussion

While self-selection of work intensity has been shown to be effective for aerobic exercise (Dishman et al., 1994; Glass & Chvala, 2001; Kravitz et al., 1997), the present study indicates that subjects do not choose a weight training intensity that is sufficient to induce strength and hypertrophic gains. Both men and women selected loads that represented only 40 to 60 % of their 1-RM, and also lifted far fewer repetitions than were expected. This was consistent across the two days of training, suggesting that the initial orientation and selection session provided no impetus to adjust training load during the subsequent bout. Interestingly, RPE data indicate subjects chose a "somewhat hard" intensity, which is similar to a number of studies of self selection during aerobic exercise (Dishman et al., 1994; Glass & Chvala, 2001; Kravitz et al., 1997; Melanson et al., 1996). Kravitz et al. (1997) had subjects complete 20 min of self selected exercise for treadmill running, simulated cross-country skiing, cycle ergometry, and aerobic riding. RPEs across modes ranged between 12.6 and 13.6.

Limited studies have examined perception of effort during resistance exercise. These studies have centered on RPE estimation during different types of resistance training (Gearhart et al., 2001; Lagally et al., 2002; O´Conner et al., 2002; Pincivero et al., 2000), or have examined state anxiety following resistance training (Bartholomew & Linder, 1998; Focht & Koltyn, 2000).

The present study employed self-selection without any prior weight training feedback or anchoring, such as a 1-RM, yet subjects selected a load similar to that seen in other studies. The perceptual cues that govern the light load selection are unknown, however it has been shown that state anxiety is reduced following resistance training at 40 - 50 % 1-RM, while anxiety is increased at heavier work loads (70 % 1-RM) (Bartholomew & Linder, 1998; Focht, 2002). Since resistance training requires that individuals overload the muscle, the intensity may be one not self selected due to the uncomfortable nature of the overload.

No gender differences were observed for relative percent 1-RM lifted, RPE and repetitions in the present study. Studies are equivocal for gender differences in RPE estimation during resistance exercise Pincivero et al. (2000) assessed isometric torque in the quadriceps muscles. Following a low anchor and high anchor test subjects completed 5 s isometric contractions ranging from 10 - 90 % MVC. Their results showed a linear increase in RPE, with no differences reported between gender. The results of the present study indicate that gender does not influence resistance training load selection, with both genders choosing a light load.

Without the use of intensity anchors (i.e. graded exercise test), research has shown that subjective regulation of effort may be ineffective. Glass and Holcomb (1997), prescribed RPEs of 11, 13 and 15 for cycling and track exercise without any prior pacing or testing to set anchors. Results showed that individuals chose intensities of 79 %, 93 % and 97 % HRR for track exercise and 72 %, 86 % and 97 % for cycle exercise at RPEs of 11, 13, and 15. These intensities far exceeded expected values, and thus cast doubt on assigning RPE intensities with no prior learning trials. On the other hand, when subjects are allowed to self select aerobic training intensity they appear to choose a relative intensity between 50 and 60 % of VO_{2max} (Dishman et al., 1994; Glass & Chvala, 2001). It has been suggested that RPE anchors be used prior to prescribing resistance training (Gearhart et al., 2001); the results of the present study suggest that future research needs to evaluate the effectiveness of learning trials on subsequent load regulation by subjects. Self-selection of weight lifting load by untrained individuals does not ensure adequate load stimulus for the development of muscular strength. Considering that strength gain is induced by overloading the muscle with a load that it is unaccustomed to, it is not surprising that perceptually, individuals were not able to select the appropriate load. While aerobic training is an activity that fall within common perceptual ranges (and thus individuals can self select accurately), resistance training is outside the typical perceptual range of effort, thus individuals cannot self select without some perceptual "training".

Practical applications

The greatest advantage of self-selected exercise is the ease of use and prospects for increased exercise adherence. By self-selecting exercise intensity, the individual needs less supervision and instruction, is more likely to increase work volume as tolerated, rather than as dictated. The results of the present study however suggest that self-selection of load intensity is not advisable for resistance training. Individuals do not appear able to choose a load that is intense enough to evoke strength and hypertrophy changes. If self-selection of weight training were used in a health and fitness environment, individuals would not notice strength gains, and would be more apt to drop out due to lack of progress. For resistance training it is essential that the trainer work with the client to perform strength testing followed by adequate instruction regarding the load required to elicit strength gains. The trainer could instruct the client regarding lifting to fatigue, appropriate repetitions and could give the client a feel for the load needed for strength gain. The client then can be trained to perceive the effort required for effective resistance training, and perhaps then they will be better able to self regulate their training. Future studies need to examine protocols to "teach" the individuals the appropriate perceptual range so that they can accurately self select resistance exercise intensity.

References

ACSM. (2000). *ACSM´s guidelines for exercise testing and prescription* (6th ed.). Lippincott: William and Wilkins.

Bartholomew, J. B., & Linder, D. E. (1998). State anxiety following resitance exercise: The role of gender and exercise intensity. *Journal of Behavioral Medicine, 21*(2), 205-219.

Borg, G. (1970). Perceived exertion as an indicator of somatic stress. *Scandinavian Journal of Rehabilitation Medicine, 2*, 92-98.

Dishman, R. K., Farquhar, R. P., & Cureton, K. J. (1994). Responses to preferred intensities of exertion in men differing in activity levels. *Medicine & Science in Sports & Exercise, 26*(6), 783-790.

Fleck, S. J., & Kraemer, W. J. (1997). *Designing resistance training programs* (2nd ed.). Champaign, IL: Human Kinetics.

Focht, B. C. (2002). Pre-exercise anxiety and the anxioletic responses to acut bouts of self-selected and prescribed intensity resistance exercise. *Journal of Sports Medicine and Physical Fitness, 42*(2), 217-223.

Focht, B. C., & Koltyn, K. A. (2000). Influence of resistance exercise of different internsities on state anxiety and blood pressure. *Journal of Sports and Exercise, 31*(3), 456-463.

Gearhart, R. E., Goss, F. L., Lagally, K. M., Jakicic, J. M., Gallagher, J., & Gallagher, K. (2001). Standardized scalling procedures for rating perceived exertion during resistance exercise. *Journal of Strength and Conditioning Research, 15*(3), 320-325.

Gearhart, R. E., Goss, F. L., Lagally, K. M., Jakicic, J. M., Gallagher, J., Gallagher, K. I., et al. (2002). Ratings of perceived exertion in active muscle during high-intensity and low-intensity resistance exercise. *Journal of Strength and Conditioning Research, 16*(1), 87-91.

Glass, S. C., & Chvala, A. M. (2001). Preferred exertion across three common modes of exercise training. *Journal of Strength and Conditioning Research, 15*(4), 474-479.

Glass, S. C., & Holcomb, R. R. (1997). Heart rate response associated with non-paced exercise prescription using ratings of perceived exertion. *Journal of Strength and Conditioning Research, 11*(4), 246-250.

Heyward, V. H. (2002). *Advanced fitness assessment & exercise prescription* (4th ed.). Champaign, IL: Human Kinetics.

Kravitz, L., Robergs, R. A., Heyward, V. H., Wagner, D. R., & Powers, K. (1997). Exercise mode and gender comparisons of energy expenditur at self-selected intensities. *Medicine & Science in Sports & Exercise, 29*(8), 1028-1035.

Lagally, K. M., Robertson, R. J., Gallagher, K. I., Goss, F. L., Jakicic, J. M., Lephart, S. M., et al. (2002). Perceived exertion, electromyography, and blood lactate during acute bouts of resistance exercise. *Medicine & Science in Sports & Exercise, 34*(3), 552-559.

Melanson, E. L., Freedson, P. S., Webb, R., Jungbluth, S., & Kozlowski, N. (1996). Exercise responses to running and in-line skating at self-selected paces. *Medicine & Science in Sports & Exercise, 28*(2), 247-250.

O´Conner, P. J., Poudevigne, M. S., & Pasley, J. D. (2002). Perceived exertion responses to novel elbow flexor eccentric action in women and men. *Medicine & Science in Sports & Exercise, 34*(5), 862-868.

Pincivero, D. M., Coelho, A. J., & Erikson, W. H. (2000). Perceived exertion during isometric quadriceps contraction. A comparison between men and women. *Journal of Sports Medicine and Physical Fitness, 40*(4), 319-326.

Pollock, M. L., Schmidt, D. H., & Jackson, A. S. (1980). Measurement of cardionrespiratory fitness and body compositiom in the clinical setting. *Comprehensive Therapy, 6*(9), 12-27.

Siri, W. E. (1961). Body composition from fluid spaces and density: analysis of methods in techniques for measuring body composition. In J. Brozek & A. Henschel (Eds.), *Techniques for measuring body composition* (pp. 223-224). Washington, D.C.: National Academy of Sciences, National Research Council.

Spelman, C. C., Pate, R. R., Macera, C. A., & Ward, D. S. (1993). Self-selected exercise intensity of habitual walkers. *Medicine & Science in Sports & Exercise, 25*(10), 1174-1179.

MICHAEL FRÖHLICH & JÜRGEN GIEßING

Muscular effort and perceived exertion in two different strength endurance training methods

Keywords: muscular effort, perceived exertion, strength endurance training, work load, prediction

Introduction

Planning training programs is generally based on determining training parameters according to the trainee's needs. Those parameters (volume, intensity, duration, and frequency of training sessions) are applied in planning resistance training programs as well as in other kinds of training programs that are aimed at improving endurance, speed or flexibility. Whereas these parameters can be considered to be objective parameters and must be considered the foundation of training programs in high performance sports, there is more emphasis on subjective criteria in recreational sports and health sports. It has been shown in various studies (Glass & Holcomb, 1997; Wanner, 1985) that using subjective criteria can be used efficiently for regulating training parameters in endurance training programs.
According to Buskies, Boeckh-Behrens and Zieschang (1996) the main advantage of using subjective criteria for regulating training parameters is that this can not only be done without any difficult kind of testing and provides immediate feedback. Rating perceived exertion (RPE) is routinely used in endurance training programs and has been proven to be an effective way of regulating training intensity, especially in recreational and health sports (cf. Borg, 2004). Buskies has dealt with the question whether this method can also be applied to resistance training programs (cf. Buskies, 1999a; Buskies, 1999b). Buskies (2001) assigned subjects to three different groups training with either "medium", "hard" or "maximum" training intensity whereas usually RPE is measured after the subject has completed the set (Gearhart et al., 2002; Hasson, Williams, & Signorile, 1989; Kraemer, Noble, Clark, & Culver, 1987; Urhausen, Schwarz, Stefan, Gabriel, & Kindermann, 2000). Most authors apply the RPE-scale developed by Borg (Borg, 1985, 2004). Borg based the RPE scale on the idea that a measure of the perceived exertion in the level of stain and/or

heaviness experienced during physical effort, as estimated by a specific rating method (cf. McGuigan, Egan, & Foster, 2004, p. 9).

Kraemer et al. (1987) used the Borg-scale in one of their studies and found a significant correlation between lactate levels and subjective RPE in nine body-builders and eight powerlifters. The authors concluded:

> „Significant increases in PRE were observed, and lactate levels did follow the perceptual responses during the exercise session (r = 0.84; p < 0.05). This observation supports the possible use of the category-ratio scale for monitoring perceptual responses in such exercise settings." (Kraemer et al., 1987, p. 251)

Suminski et al. (1997) studied metabolic and cardiovascular reactions to strength training as well as RPE in eight male subjects doing seven strength training exercises at 50 % and 70 % of their 1-RM. Whereas RPE has been shown to be useful in strength training programs of recreational trainees, there is a lack of findings concerning its use for elite trainee who compete on a national or international level.

As a consequence of this lack of data, this study was designed in order to provide empirical data on the question whether there is a significant correlation between relative training intensity and RPE for elite trainees using two different kinds of training methods.

Materials and methods

Subjects

The 39 subjects participating in this study consisted of 13 subjects who had no strength training experience and participated in sports only on a recreational level (UN), 13 elite track and field athletes (AT) and 13 elite wrestlers (WR). Subjects in the AT and WR groups had been competing on a national or international level for seven to ten years and had been using strength training programs as a part of their training for several years as well. Table 1 shows the amount of time per week that subjects had been regularly devoting to strength training before the study was conducted. The physiological and anthropometric characteristics of the subjects population are presented in table 2.

Table 1: Absolute frequency and percent value of strength training volume (hours per week) for the untrained men (UN), athletes (AT) and the wrestlers (WR) (cf. Fröhlich, 2003, p. 84)

hours per week	UN	AT	WR
1 - 3 h	1 (100 %)	5 (38.5 %)	7 (53.8 %)
3 - 5 h		5 (38.5 %)	5 (38.5 %)
5 - 7 h		1 (7.7 %)	1 (7.7 %)
7 - 10 h		2 (15.4 %)	

Table 2: Subjects structural dimensions descriptives as well as 1-RM in bench press performance by the two different strength training settings. UN = untrained men, AT = athletes, WR = wrestlers

	age [yrs]	height [cm]	weight [kg]	1-RM [kg] T1	1-RM [kg] T2
UN	35.4 ± 7.6	179.5 ± 5.7	76.3 ± 5.7	70.0 ± 10.1	70.0 ± 10.1
AT	26.1 ± 7.6	183.5 ± 10.0	84.6 ± 14.7	105.4 ± 22.1	105.6 ± 21.4
WR	25.3 ± 10.6	175.0 ± 8.8	77.9 ± 16.1	94.0 ± 16.4	93.9 ± 16.4

Conceptual formulation

After completing two standardised training sessions in order to accustom subjects to the training method "constant load" consisting of six sets of bench presses at 60 % of 1-RM on a regular smith machine subjects were asked to complete as many repetitions as possible (cf. Fröhlich, Schmidtbleicher, Emrich, & Coen, 2003). The training method "constant number of repetitions" was based upon a test that individually determined the resistance that subjects could lift for 20-RM. Breaks between sets were 60 seconds for both training methods. By determining the range of motion over which the weight was lifted the criteria "physical work" could be calculated for each set (Fröhlich, Klein, Emrich, & Schmidtbleicher, 2001). The second testing session was done exactly one week after the first one (Oschütz, 1991). Immediately after determining 1-RM as well as after each set the subjects' RPE were noted down. The rest between determining 1-RM and the first set was three minutes in all cases.

Statistical procedure

All data was entered in the STATISTICA 5.1 statistical analysis software program. Mean and standard deviation data was presented for all subject characteristics. Percent and frequency curve was calculated. One way analysis of variance (ANOVA) and Scheffé post hoc testing were used to identify significant differences among the groups. Paired t-tests were used to evaluate the differences between the two different training settings. Two way analysis of variance (ANOVA) with repeated measurements was used to evaluate differences between groups and series. Pearson´s product moment correlation was used to examine the relationship between 1-RM, work load and RPE. An alpha level less than or equal to 0.05 was required for statistical significance.

Results

There was a highly significant difference between maximal concentric strength of the subjects in the three groups for the training method "constant number of repetitions" [$F_{(2; 36)} = 15.40$; $p < 0,05$] as well as for the training method "constant load" [$F_{(2; 36)} = 14.77$; $p < 0.05$]. Post hoc single case comparisons showed that the results of the untrained subjects were significantly different from those of the wrestlers [$p < 0.05$] and the athletes [$p < 0.05$] (cf. Fröhlich 2003) for both training methods. Within the groups of elite wrestlers and athletes there were no significant differences, neither was there a significant difference between the results of the first testing session compared to the second one. Figure 1 shows the subjects' RPE after determining 1-RM. 59 % of the subjects in the "constant load" group rated the effort during their 1-RM test as "very hard" or "very, very hard". In the other group ("constant number of repetitions") the percentage was even lower (41 %, see table 3).

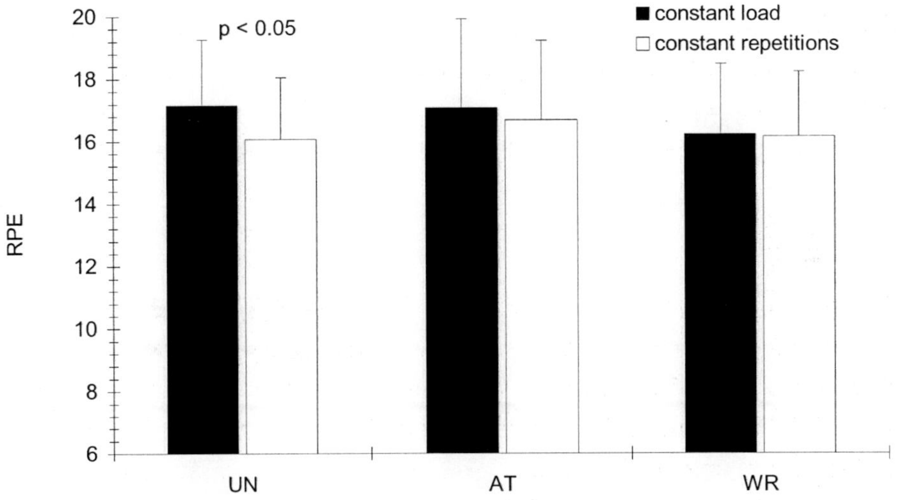

Figure 1: RPE by UN (= untrained men), AT (= athletes) and WR (= wrestlers) in 1-RM tests in the two different strength endurance training methods (left: "constant load", right: "constant repetitions")

Table 3: Absolute frequency and percent of the RPE in 1-RM tests by the two different strength training methods ("constant load", "constant repetitions")

	strength training method „constant load"		**strength training method "constant repetitions"**	
	frequency	percent	frequency	percent
12	1	2.6	-	-
somewhat hard	3	7.7	4	10.3
14	1	2.6	2	5.1
hard	9	23.1	13	33.3
16	2	5.1	4	10.3
very hard	8	20.5	3	7.7
18	4	10.3	6	15.4
very, very hard	3	7.7	2	5.1
20	8	20.5	5	12.8

Results show no significant correlation between maximum concentric strength and RPE [r = -0.16; p = 0.30; N = 39] for the training method „constant load" and [r = 0.16; p = 0.30; N = 39] for subjects in the group that trained with a constant number of repetitions. The results of the three groups were as follows: Training method "constant load": UN [r = 0.02; p = 0.95]; AT [r = -0.52; p = 0.07] and WR [r = 0.24; p = 0.42]. Training method "constant number of repetitions": UN [r = -0.31; p = 0.30]; AT [r = 0.08; p = 0.80] and WR [r = 0.48; p = 0.10]. Figure 2 and 3 show the work load as well as the RPE in the six sets for the two different strength endurance training methods "constant load" and "constant number of repetitions".

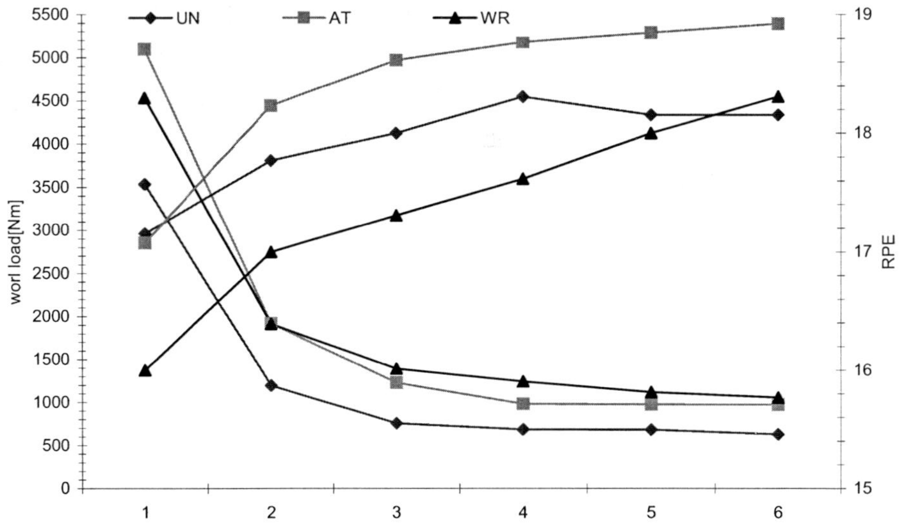

Figure 2: Work load [Nm] and RPE over six sets in untrained men (UN), athletes (AT) and wrestlers (WR) for the strength endurance training method "constant load"

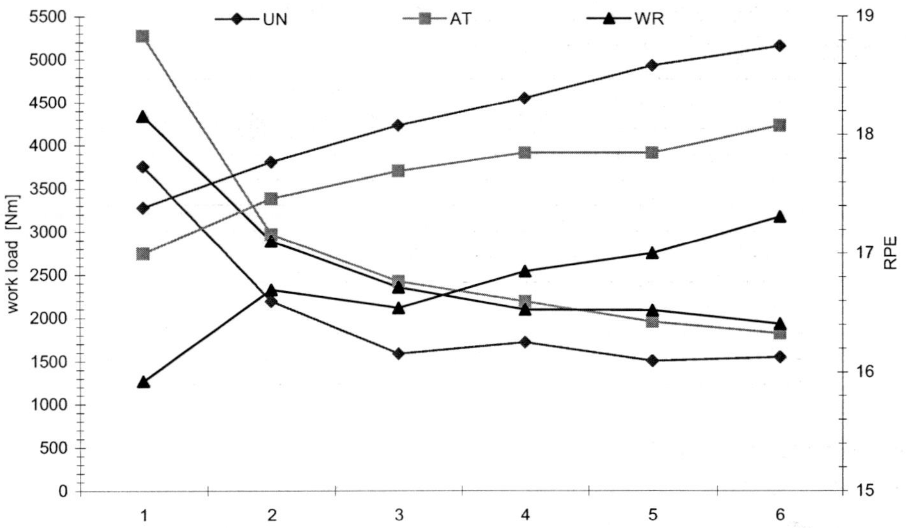

Figure 3: Work load [Nm] and RPE over six sets in untrained men (UN), athletes (AT) and wrestlers (WR) for the strength endurance training method "constant number of repetitions" (20-RM)

There is no significant correlation between work load and PRE over the sets in the strength training method "constant load" (cf. figure 4). The only exception is the significant correlation in the group of UN in the first set [$r = 0.86$; $p < 0.05$]. In the strength training method "constant repetition" (20-RM) there is a significant correlation between work load and RPE in the fourth set [$r = 0.61$; $p < 0.05$], the fifth set [$r = 0.63$; $p < 0.05$] and the sixth set [$r = .67$; $p < 0.05$] in the group of UN, as well as in the AT group in the fourth set [$r = 0.60$; $p < 0.05$] and in the sixth sets [$r = 0.56$; $p < 0.05$]. In addition to that, a negative significant correlation between work load and RPE in the second set [$r = -0.65$; $p < 0.05$] in the WR group was found.

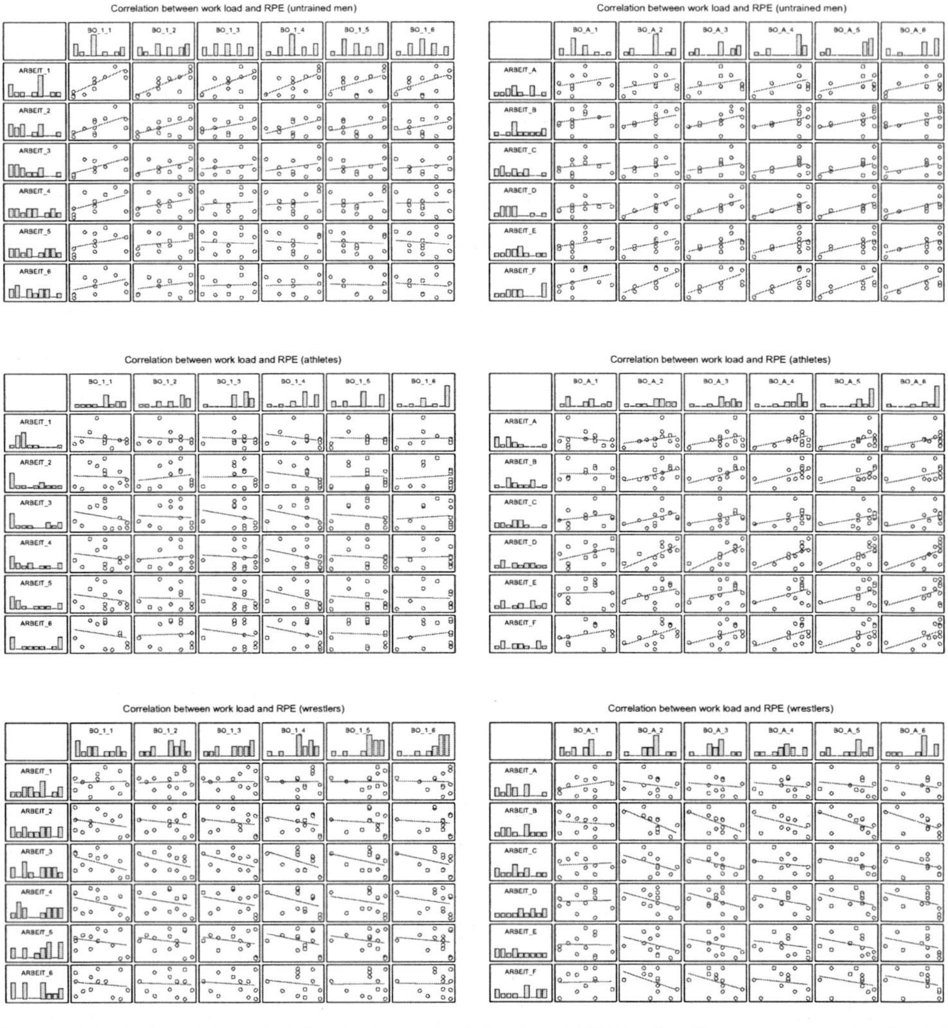

Figure 4: Matrixplot of the correlation between work load and RPE in the different groups. On the left: training method for "constant load" (60 % 1-RM), on the right: training method for "constant repetitions" (20-RM)

Discussion and conclusion

Several studies have shown that RPE can be successfully applied to determine intensity of endurance training programs (cf. Borg, 2004). However, research analysing if this also applies to resistance training programs is scarce. Some suggestions have been made by Buskies and colleagues (1996) who used a categorisation that asked subjects to either perform their sets at "medium", "high" or "maximum" intensity. In our study subjects reported their RPE immediately after completing their set. Neither for the training method "constant load" nor for the training method "constant number of repetitions" a significant correlation between RPE and other factors studied could be found. Furthermore it is remarkable that although wrestlers could realise more repetitions at 60 % of 1-RM as well as a higher "physical work" and load for the sets three to six of "constant load" compared to the other groups, their RPE was less than that of athletes and untrained subjects. One possible explanation for this phenomenon could be the fact that strength endurance training is usually a vital part of the wrestlers' training programs. Therefore, wrestlers are usually accustomed to the pain that results from an accumulation of lactate and are consequently desensitized accordingly. This explanation is in accordance with findings by Lecsko and Varisco (1999) who found a higher pain threshold during a strength endurance training program in trained subjects compared to untrained subjects.

Kraemer et al. (1987) had nine bodybuilders and eight power-lifters perform three sets for 10-RM of ten different exercises (bench press, double leg extensions, shoulder press, double leg curl, upright row, leg press, lat pull down, sated calf raises, two-arm curls und hang cleans) and found significant correlations ($r = 0.84$) between lactate levels and RPE.

Suminski et al. (1997) had subjects do 7 different exercises at 50 % of 1-RM and 70 % of 1-RM and found that RPE corresponded with lactate levels but not with heart rate and blood pressure. Hasson et al. (1989) found a significant correlation [$r = 0.49$ to 0.89, $p = 0.05$] between root mean squared EMG and RPE as well as an inverse correlation of mean power frequency of EMG and RPE:

> "In summary, the results of this investigation indicate that during sustained isometric exercise leading to exhaustion, changes in the perception of effort are related to changes in both the amplitude and frequency content of the EMG signal." (Hasson et al., 1989, p. 102)

Pierce, Rozenek and Stone (1993) found a significant reduction of lactate acid concentration (LA), heart rate (HR), and rating of perceived exertion as an expression of training adaptation after eight weeks of "high volume weight training" (the experimental group trained twice a day, three times a week, training consisted of 3 weeks of 3 x 10 RM, followed by 3 weeks of 3 x 5 RM, followed by 2 weeks of 3 x 10 RM). The authors deduced by the results:

> "...that an 8-week, high volume weight training program results in beneficial effects on (La) HR, and RPE responses to weight training exercise at an absolute load (Repetitions x Weight)." (Pierce et al., 1993, p. 213)

Buskies (2001, p. 57) considers RPE to be an appropriate parameter for planning resistance training programs. Urhausen et al. (2000) suggests that RPE is not suitable for patients who use strength training as a part of physical therapy. Those suggestions, however, can not be generalised for all weight trainers. It must also be taken into consideration that there is a huge difference between the needs of people who weight train on a recreational level or as a part of physical therapy and those who compete at national or international levels and use weight training as a part of their training regimen (cf. McGuigan et al., 2004).

In our study the Borg-scale was used and RPE was determined immediately after completion of each set. A posteriori calculations showed that there were no significant correlations between physical work and RPE. Neither for the two training methods used nor for any of the three groups of subjects tested in this study RPE correlated significantly with objective criteria like work load or number of repetitions. These results demonstrate that although RPE might be useful as a valid criteria for designing resistance training programs on a recreational level as some authors have suggested, RPE failed to prove its effectiveness for the training methods and groups of subjects observed in this study.

References

Borg, G. (1985). Psychophysical studies of effort and exertion: some historical, theoretical and empirical aspects. In G. Borg & D. Ottoson (Eds.), *The perception of exertion in physical work* (pp. 3-12). Basingstroke: Macmillan.

Borg, G. (2004). Anstrengungsempfinden und körperliche Aktivität [Perceived exertion and physical activity]. *Deutsches Ärzteblatt, 101*(15), A1016-A1021.

Buskies, W. (1999a). Sanftes Krafttraining nach dem subjektiven Belastungsempfinden versus Training bis zur muskulären Ausbelastung [Moderate strength training regulated by RPE versus training until muscle exhaustion]. *Deutsche Zeitschrift für Sportmedizin, 50*(10), 316-320.

Buskies, W. (1999b). *Sanftes Krafttraining. Unter besonderer Berücksichtigung des subjektiven Belastungsempfindens [Moderate strength training. Under special consideration of the rate of perceived exertion]*. Köln: Sport und Buch Strauß.

Buskies, W. (2001). Zur Bedeutung des sanften Krafttrainings nach dem subjektiven Belastungsempfinden [The importance of moderate strength training regulated by RPE]. *Sportwissenschsaft, 31*(1), 45-60.

Buskies, W., Boeckh-Behrens, W.-U., & Zieschang, K. (1996). Möglichkeiten der Intensitätssteuerung im gesundheitsorientierten Krafttraining [Regulation of intensity in health-orientated strength training]. *Sportwissenschaft, 26*(2), 170-183.

Fröhlich, M. (2003). *Kraftausdauertraining. Eine empirische Studie zur Methodik [Strength endurance training. An empirical study]*. Göttingen: Cuvillier.

Fröhlich, M., Klein, M., Emrich, E., & Schmidtbleicher, D. (2001). Arbeit als Bruttokriterium der Belastung im Kraftausdauertraining [Work as gross criterium of the work load in strength endurance training]. *Leistungssport, 31*(2), 24-28.

Fröhlich, M., Schmidtbleicher, D., Emrich, E., & Coen, B. (2003). Metabolische und kardiovaskuläre Beanspruchung bei spezifisch trainierten und untrainierten Männern im Kraftausdauertraining [Metabolic and cardiovascular response in specifically trained and untrained males in strength endurance training]. *Deutsche Zeitschrift für Sportmedizin, 54*(12), 355-360.

Gearhart, R. E., Goss, F. L., Lagally, K. M., Jakicic, J. M., Gallagher, J., Gallagher, K. I., et al. (2002). Ratings of perceived exertion in active muscle during high-intensity and low-intensity resistance exercise. *Journal of Strength and Conditioning Research, 16*(1), 87-91.

Glass, S. C., & Holcomb, R. R. (1997). Heart rate response associated with non-paced exercise prescription using ratings of perceived exertion. *Journal of Strength and Conditioning Research, 11*(4), 246-250.

Hasson, S. M., Williams, J. H., & Signorile, J. F. (1989). Fatigue-induced changes in myoelectric signal characteristics and perceived exertion. *Canadian Journal of Sports Science, 14*(2), 99-102.

Kraemer, W. J., Noble, B. J., Clark, M. J., & Culver, B. W. (1987). Physiologic responses to heavy-resistance exercise with very short rest periods. *International Journal of Sports Medicine, 8*(4), 247-252.

Lecsko, S., & Varisco, F. (1999). Kardiovaskuläre und metabolische Beanspruchung beim Krafttraining. Ein Vergleich der physiologischen Parameter Blutdruck, Herzfrequenz und Blutlaktat vor, während und nach einem Kraftausdauertraining [Cardiovascular and metabolic response during strength training. Comparison of blood pressure, heart rate before, during and after strength endurance training]. *Physiotherapie, 4*, 19-28.

McGuigan, M. R., Egan, A. D., & Foster, C. (2004). Salivary cortisol responses and perceived exertion during high intensity and low intensity bouts of resistance exercise. *Journal of Sports Science and Medicine, 3*(1), 8-15.

Oschütz, H. (1991). Chronobiologie im Sport - Zur Entwicklung der sportlichen Leistungsfähigkeit unter Berücksichtigung der Cirkadian-Rhythmik [Chronobiology in sports -

the development of sport performance under consideration of circadian-rhythmicity]. *Leistungssport, 21*(4), 12-15.

Pierce, K., Rozenek, R., & Stone, H. M. (1993). Effects of high volume weight training on lactate, heart rate, and perceived exertion. *Journal of Strength and Conditioning Research, 7*(4), 211-215.

Suminski, R. R., Robertson, R. J., Arslanian, S., Kang, J., Utter, A. C., DaSilvio, S. G., et al. (1997). Perception of effort during resistance exercise. *Journal of Strength and Conditioning Research, 11*(4), 261-265.

Urhausen, A., Schwarz, M., Stefan, S., Gabriel, H., & Kindermann, W. (2000). Kardiovaskuläre und metabolische Beanspruchung durch einen Kraftausdauer-Zirkel in der ambulanten Herztherapie [Cardiovascular and metabolic strain during a strength-endurance circle training in out-patient cardiac rehabilitation]. *Deutsche Zeitschrift für Sportmedizin, 51*(4), 130-136.

Wanner, H.-U. (1985). Subjektive Einstufung der Belastung bei Ausdauerleistungen [Subjective classification of exertion in endurance performance]. *Deutsche Zeitschrift für Sportmedizin, 36*(4), 104-112.

NIKLAS LICHTENEGGER

The relationship between myostatin function, strength gain and muscle hypertrophy

Keywords: myostatin function, muscle hypertrophy, growth hormone, gen expression, relationship

Introduction

Inasmuch as the study of literature tries to document the interaction of exercise and growth hormone (GH), testosterone and the expression of various muscle-specific genes, a detailed discussion of the issues involved is warranted (Lichtenegger, 2000). Control of growth hormone and testosterone release during muscular exercise and the expression of various muscle-specific genes like myostatin is a challenging question not yet elucidated in spite of the numerous studies.

Several attempts have been made to characterize the events leading to increase in muscle mass and strength (Häkkinen, Komi, Alen, & Kauhanen, 1987) and there is no doubt that resistance exercise is a potent stimulus for muscle tissue hypertrophy and strength development (Kraemer et al., 1991).

It seems to be obvious that the limited potential for strength development in elite athletes and the magnitude of hypertrophic adaptations cannot be compared with the possible training adaptations for untrained subjects, but as demonstrated by Häkkinen et al. (1987), the basic neuromuscular mechanisms increasing strength during training among elite-athletes might not differ from those for less-trained individuals, only the initial trained status of the athletes makes the process more difficult to substantiate.

Heavy-resistance exercise has been shown to produce an acute burst of serum anabolic hormones of testosterone, free testosterone and growth hormone. The relatively largest acute hormone responses have been observed after the hypertrophic type of strength training session (Sallinen et al., 2004).

As resistance training is accompanied by muscle damage and regenerative processes, which leads to various remodeling processes, Sorichter, Puschendorf and Mair (1999) reported a cascade of reactions which resulted in an activated skeletal muscle protein metabolism.

Fiatarone-Singh et al. (1999) suggested that such muscle damage is a step in remodeling processes that leads to muscle regeneration. Willoughby and Taylor (2004a) found that it is conceivable that the consistent elevations in serum testosterone after each exercise bout mediated the up-regulation in androgen receptor expression, which subsequently led to an enhanced ligand-binding capacity and a concomitant increase in myofibrillar protein and that heavy resistance training possibly increases myofibrillar protein content by way of the androgen-receptors signalling pathway.

To enhance the development of muscular strength and size with heavy resistance training, optimal conditions for recovery are necessary. This recovery period is accompanied by a host of influences including the actions of specific hormones, nutrient intake, sleep and many other factors. Houston (1999) described the interaction of an appropriate combination of diet, resistance exercise training and rest, in order to gain muscle mass, as an endogenous system regulating the mass of skeletal muscle.

In fact, quantitative estimates suggest that about 1 - 2 % of all skeletal muscle is synthesized and broken down daily. Both synthesis and breakdown are controlled by cellular mechanisms that include the activation of gene transcription, initiation of protein synthesis, and several proteolytic enzyme pathways (Rasmussen & Phillips, 2003). Viru, Smirnova, Karelson, Snegovskaya and Viru (1996) mentioned that growth hormone, testosterone and even thyroid hormones can interact with protein synthesis in the muscle. They thereby promote training effects on muscle fibers. It is generally accepted that, possibly mediated through these hormones (among other factors), body protein is in a continuous state of turnover, with new proteins being synthesized and old ones degraded.

In addition, hormonal changes are induced by training sessions (Viru, Litvinova, Smirnova, & Viru, 1994) and the hormones that can influence protein synthesis also include insulin and insulin-like growth factor-I (IGF-I) (Chandler, Byrne, Patterson, & Ivy, 1994). As Kraemer, Kilgore, Kraemer and Castracane (1992) reported that growth hormone promotes protein synthesis by facilitating the transport of amino acids.

It has been well shown that basal concentrations of anabolic hormones are influenced by total energy and nutrient intake (Forbes, Brown, Welle, & Underwood, 1989; Longtrope, Feldman, McKinlay, & Araujo, 2000; Volek, Kraemer, Bush, Incledon, & Boetes, 1997). Forbes et al. (1989) reported that three weeks overfeeding caused an increases in the plasma level of testosterone, insulin-like growth factor-1 (IGF-1) and insulin. Various studies have shown that elevated serum testosterone increases androgen receptors in proliferating myoblasts (Phillips, Tipton, Aarsland, Wolf, & Wolfe, 1997) and may be associated with elevated myofibrillar protein synthesis (Willoughby & Taylor, 2004b). The results of Sallinen et al. (2004) suggest that dietary fat and protein intake may lead to alterations in the regulation of the endocrine system during prolonged strength training.

Although Volek et al. (1997) showed that percent energy of protein was negatively correlated with serum pre-exercise testosterone concentrations in male strength athletes, it seems likely, that there are stronger factors than the diet that regulate growth hormone secretion after the exercise e.g., metabolic byproducts, body composition, fitness status, hormones and growth factors, thus heavy-resistance exercise (HRE) suggest that the moderate intake of both fat and protein could be recommended for strength athletes (Sallinen et al., 2004). Since muscle mass, especially cross-sectional areas of the muscle, and muscle strength are two strongly related characteristic, more muscle mass would implicate (in part) more strength (Huygens et al., 2004).

The role of hormone regulation may become increasingly important for muscle hypertrophy and strength development in strength athletes with a long and intense training background (Ahtiainen, Pakarinen, Alen, Kraemer, & Hakkinen, 2003). Myostatin (Growth and Differentiation Factor 8 or GDF-8) is a member of the transforming growth factor ß (TGF-ß) superfamily of secreted growth and differentiation factors that is essential for proper regulation of skeletal muscle (McPherron & Lee, 1997), acts as a negative regulator of skeletal muscle mass (Huygens et al., 2004) and is a catabolic regulator of skeletal muscle via proteolytic and atrophic mechanisms (Willoughby & Taylor, 2004a). Myostatin is a secreted negative regulator of skeletal muscle growth, hence its role in muscle wasting is being investigated in various laboratories (Sharma, Langley, Bass, & Kambadur, 2001), because how myostatin influences muscle phenotypes is unclear (Roth et al., 2003). Higher levels of myostatin immunoreactivity have been reported in the muscle and serum of HIV-infected men with muscle wasting (Gonzalez-Cadavid et al., 1998).

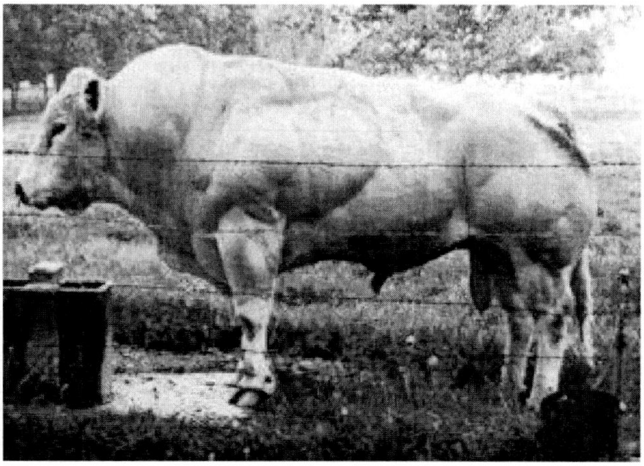

Figure 1: Belgien Blue cattle (Hertrampf, Matsakas, Friedl, Seibl, & Diel, 2004)

Such observations indicate that the level of circulating myostatin may have a role in regulating changes in muscle size (Walker, Kambadur, Sharma, & Smith, 2004). However the proteins that facilitate myostatin secretion and the latency complex of myostatin are not yet characterized (Sharma et al., 2001). Mutations in the coding sequence of bovine myostatin are known to have increases in muscle mass. McPherron and Lee (1997) reported about the myostatin sequences and the identification of mutations in the coding sequence of bovine myostatin in two breeds of double-muscled cattle, Belgian Blue (figure 1) and Piedmontese, which are known to have an increase in muscle mass relative to conventional cattle.

Individual muscles in myostatin null mice weigh 2- to 3-fold more than those of wild-type mice (figure 2), primarily due to an increased number of muscle fibers without a corresponding increase in the amount of fat (McPherron & Lee, 1997). Thus myostatin-null mutant mice have both muscle hyperplasia and hypertrophy, which can be related to increased satellite cell activity, and myostatin may function as an inhibitor of satellite cell proliferation (Sharma et al., 2001).

The increase of muscle mass resulted from muscle cell hyperplasia and hypertrophy (McPherron & Lee, 1997), which suggests that myostatin is a negative regulator of muscle growth (Sharma et al., 2001). The muscular hypertrophy which has been observed in many breeds of cattle, appears to be inherited as a single major autosomal locus with several modifiers of phenotypic expression, resulting in incomplete penetrance (Ménissier, 1982). The mutation,

which is partially recessive, causes an average increase in muscle mass of 20 - 25 %, a decrease in mass of most other organs and a decrease in intramuscular fat and connective tissue (Hanset, 1982).
However, whether myostatin regulates skeletal muscle mass in humans in the same way as in nonhumans species is unclear (Huygens et al., 2004).

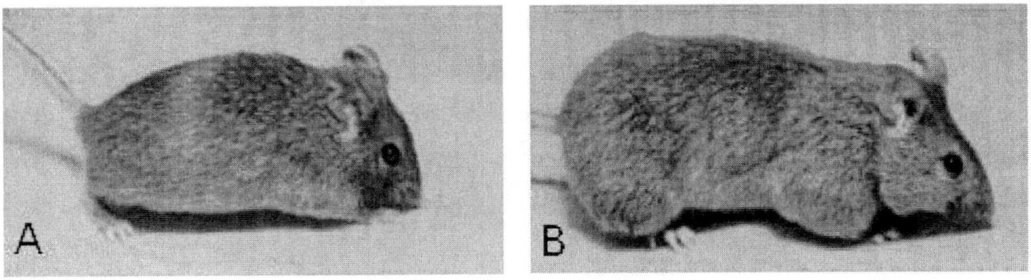

Figure 2: A) wild type mouse, B) myostatin null mouse (adapted from Hertrampf et al., 2004)

Muscle size is considered to be one of the most heritable quantitative traits in humans, with genetic variation accounting for as much as 92 % - 94 % of the total variance in muscle circumference (Ferrell et al., 1999).
In addition to skeletal muscle, low levels of myostatin have been found in adipose tissue (McPherron, Lawler, & Lee, 1997) and has been suggested to inhibit preadipocyte (Sharma et al., 2001). Myostatin gene expression appears to be transcriptionally regulated during myogenesis, in postnatal muscle, and in response to some physiological conditions in adults (Sharma et al., 2001). Myostatin has also been hypothesized to play a role in the muscle regeneration process. Following skeletal muscle injury, the degeneration process, such as inflammation, neutrophil infiltration, and macrophage phagocytosis of neurotic cells, occurs within the damaged region. This process is then followed by the activation of satellite cells, which exist in skeletal muscle in a quiescent stat. Activated satellite cells proliferate and migrate to the site of injury where they fuse to form myotubes and mature into skeletal muscle fibers (Sharma et al., 2001).
Although the function of myostatin in early myogenesis is well established, its role in the adult muscle is poorly understood (Sharma et al., 2001) and the identification of significantly linked genes might allow us to identify the variations in coding sequences at the genomic level responsible for the interindividual phenotypic variation in skeletal muscle mass and strength (Huygens et al., 2004). Unfortunately, studies to date examining myostatin in skeletal mus-

cle regeneration are correlative and do not show a direct causative role for myostatin in muscle regeneration after injury (Sharma et al., 2001).
Huygens et al. (2004) showed in a literature overview that myostatin has an important functional role in muscle mass of mice and cattle, that myostatin blockers have positive effects on muscle growth, and that linkage studies on muscularity in humans are lacking. Moreover, Huygens et al. (2004) showed that in this first explorative linkage study in humans to see whether the myostatin pathway might explain interindividual differences in estimated muscle cross-sectional area and knee strength, the findings suggest that the chromosomal regions 2q32.2, 6p21.2 and 13q14.2 might harbor potential quantitative trait loci (QTLs) for skeletal muscle strength with myostatin (GDF8), CDKN1A, and MYOD1 as good candidate genes.
Consequently, muscle immobilisation increases the expression of myostatin whereas subsequent muscle re-loading results in decreases in myostatin expression (Wehling, Cai, & Tidball, 2000). Roth et al. (2003) observed a significant decrease in myostatin expression in response to 9 weeks of heavy-resistance strength training in previously sedentary, healthy men and women (figure 3).

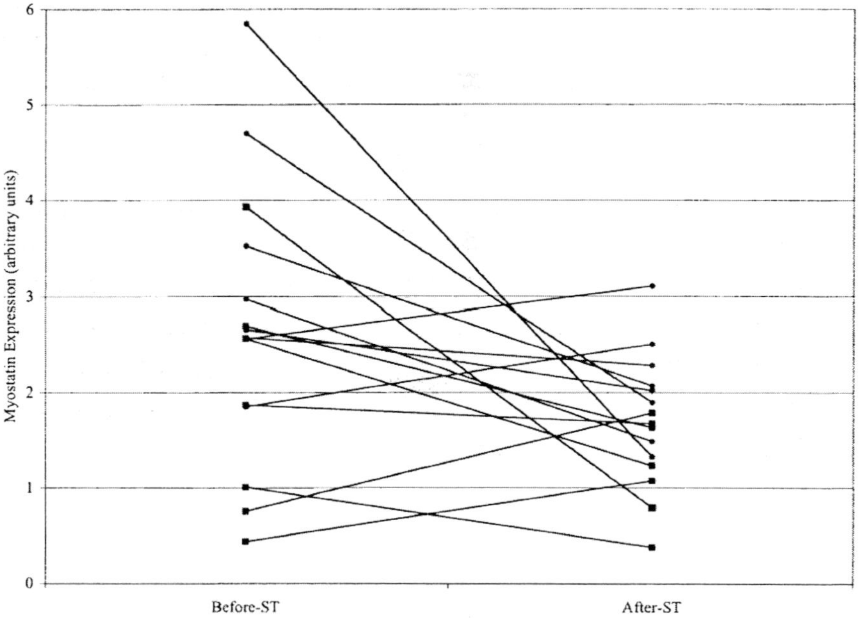

Figure 3: Myostatin expression levels (arbitrary units) for before strength training (ST) (n= 15) versus after ST (n = 15) for each individual. •, males; ■, females. A significant decrease in myostatin expression was observed in response to ST, p<0.05, with no group differences. (Roth et al., 2003)

Therefore strength training reduces skeletal muscle myostatin expression in sedentary, healthy men and women and these data provide evidence that myostatin is responsive to muscle loading in healthy adult humans, with no age or gender differences which may have relevance in future work where myostatin is studied as a therapeutic target for muscle wasting disorders (Roth et al., 2003).

The mechanism by which myostatin inhibits muscle growth is uncertain, although Sharma et al. (2001) have suggested an inhibitory effect on skeletal muscle satellite cells. Thus, myostatin expression appears responsive to elevated glucocorticoids (Ma et al., 2003) and muscle immobilisation/inactivity (Carlson, Booth, & Gordon, 1999; Wehling et al., 2000; Willoughby, Sultemeire, & Brown, 2003).

In contrast, IGF-1 (Walker et al., 2004), testosterone and human growth hormone are known to be positive modulators of muscle growth. Also, some genes encoding proteins that play an important role in myogenesis (e.g., myogenin, IGF-1) did not show signs of linkage to explain variation in muscle mass or strength (Huygens et al., 2004) (figure 4).

These findings go together with these of Walker et al. (2004) although they attempt that local muscle IGF-1 appears to be more important than circulating levels to increases in muscle size with resistance training. Myostatin may play a role in exercise-induced increases in muscle size, its circulating levels decreasing with training (Walker et al., 2004).

Even in earlier studies, without the possibility of gaining myostatin levels following strength training protocols, Reis, Frick and Schmidtbleicher (1995) established a systems model of training following the follicular and the luteal phase in women and attempted that training taking the regular endocrine changes during the menstrual cycle into consideration seems to reveal new resources in females training adaptations These findings based on hormone concentrations of the sexual hormone binding globulin (SHBG) and, among others, Testosterone and cortisol.

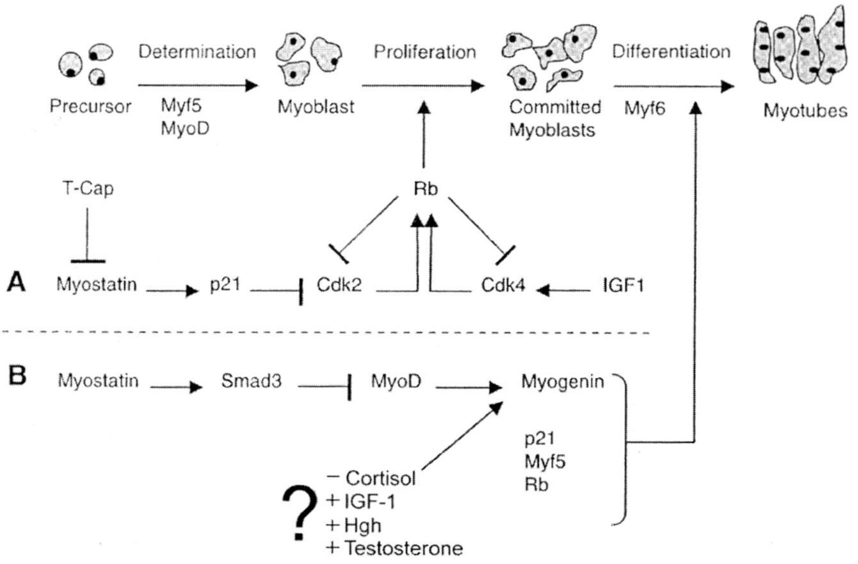

Figure 4: An adapted model from Langley et al., 2002 (in Huygens et al., 2004) for the role of myostatin and IGF-1 in mitotic (A) and myogenic (B) conditions. Myf5 and MyoD specify cells to the myogenin control myoblast differention. ***A:*** *in growing medium, myostatin upregulates p21, an inhibitor of Cdk2, which results in hypophosphorylation of Rb and cell cycle arrest of proliferating myoblasts. Titin-cap can bind to myostatin and block its secretion. IGF-1 stimulates myoblast proliferation by Cdk4 and hyperphosphorylation of Rb.* ***B:*** *in myogenic medium, myostatin represses the levels of MyoD, myogenin, p21, and Myf5 via Smad3-MyoD interaction, leading to the inhibition of myoblast differentiation. Decreased levels of MyoD lead to decreased binding with Rb and improper cell cycle withdrawal. In contrast IGF-1 induces differentiation via upregulating Myf5 and myogenin. Arrows = stimulating, block-endet lines = inhibiting. (Modificated by Lichtenegger, 2005)*

In addition, enhanced stimulation of growth hormone secretion by testosterone increases the production of IGF via GH-mediated mechanisms and may also help produce various anabolic properties (Kraemer, 1992). Could it therefore be assumed, that these previous findings about the various hormonal functions have influence on the negative growth and differentiating factor myostatin, such as Walker et al. (2004) indicated that IGF-1 may have a role in regulating myostatin function (figure 4)?

To establish a new systems model of training depending on this findings, further research is needed to shed light on the numerous and complex physiological mechanisms contributing to resistance exercise performance decrements as far as further studies with specific protocols are needed to confirm if the myostatin function and response could be an indicator of the timing of adaptations to training.

References

Ahtiainen, J. P., Pakarinen, A., Alen, M., Kraemer, W. J., & Hakkinen, K. (2003). Muscle hypertrophy, hormonal adaptations and strength development during strength training in strength-trained and untrained men. *European Journal of Applied Physiology, 89*(6), 555-563.

Carlson, C. J., Booth, F. W., & Gordon, S. E. (1999). Skeletal muscle myostatin mRNA expression is fiber-type specific and increases during hindlimb unloading. *American Journal of Physiology, 277*(40), R601-R606.

Chandler, R. M., Byrne, H. K., Patterson, J. G., & Ivy, J. L. (1994). Dietary supplements affect the anabolic hormones after weight-training exercise. *Journal of Applied Physiology, 76*(2), 839-845.

Ferrell, R. E., Conte, V., Lawrence, E. C., Roth, S. M., Hagberg, J. M., & Hurley, B. F. (1999). Frequent sequence variation in the human myostatin (GDF8) gene as a marker for analysis of muscle-related phenotypes. *Genomics, 62*(2), 203-207.

Fiatorone-Singh, M. A., Ding, W., Manfredi, T. J., Solares, G. S., Neill, E. F., Clements, K. M., et al. (1999). Insulin like growth factor I in skeletal muscle after weight-lifting exercise in frail elders. *American Journal of Physiology, 277*(40), E135-E143.

Forbes, G. B., Brown, M. R., Welle, S. L., & Underwood, L. E. (1989). Hormonal response to overfeeding. *American Journal of Clinical Nutrition, 49*(4), 608-611.

Gonzalez-Cadavid, N. F., Taylor, W. E., Yarasheski, K., Sinha-Hikim, I., Ma, K., Ezzat, S., et al. (1998). Organization of the human myostatin gene and expression in healthy men and HIV-infected men with muscle wasting. *Proceedings of the National Academy of Sciences of the United States of America, 95*(25), 14938-14943.

Häkkinen, K., Komi, P. V., Alen, M., & Kauhanen, H. (1987). EMG, muscle fibre and force production characteristics during a 1 year training period in elite weight-lifters. *European Journal of Applied Physiology and Occupational Physiology, 56*(4), 419-427.

Hanset, R. (1982). Muscle hypertrophy of genetic origin and its use to omprove beef production. In F. Menissier (Ed.), *The Hague*. The Netherlands: Nijhoff.

Hertrampf, T., Matsakas, A., Friedl, A., Seibl, J., & Diel, P. (2004). Der Wachstumsfaktor Myostatin [The growth factor myostatin]. *f.i.t. das Wissenschaftsmagazin der Deutschen Sporthochschule Köln, 1*(9), 8-11.

Houston, M. E. (1999). Gaining weight: The scientific basis of increasing skeletal muscle mass. *Canadian Journal of Applied Physiology, 24(4)*, 305-316.

Huygens, W., Thomis, M. A., Peeters, M. W., Aerssens, J., Janssen, R., Vlietinck, R. F., et al. (2004). Linkage of myostatin pathway genes with knee strength in humans. *Physiology Genomics, 17*(3), 264-270.

Kraemer, W. J. (1992). Hormonal mechanims related to the expression of muscular strength and power. In P. V. Komi (Ed.), *Strength and power in sport* (pp. 64-76). Oxford: Blackwell Scientific Publications.

Kraemer, W. J., Gordon, S. E., Fleck, S. J., Marchitelli, L. J., Mello, R., Dziados, J. E., et al. (1991). Endogenous anabolic hormonal and growth factor responses to heavy resistance exercise in males and females. *International Journal of Sports Medicine, 12*(2), 228-235.

Kraemer, W. J., Kilgore, J. L., Kraemer, G. R., & Castracane, V. D. (1992). Growth hormone, IGF-I, and testosterone responses to resistitive exercise. *Medicine & Science in Sports & Exercise, 24*(12), 1346-1353.

Lichtenegger, N. (2000). *An alternative systems model of training under admission of natural endocrine function and especially considering human growth hormone*. Karl-Franzens Graz: Institut of Sports Sciences (unpublished).

Longtrope, C., Feldman, H. A., McKinlay, J. B., & Araujo, A. B. (2000). Diet and sex hormone-binding globulin. *Journal of Clinical Endocrinology and Metabolism, 85*, 293-296.

Ma, K., Mallidis, C., Bhasin, S., Mahabadi, V., Artaza, J., Gonzalez-Cavidad, N., et al. (2003). Glucocorticoid-induced skeletal muscle atrophy is associated with up-regulation of myostatin gene expression. *American Journal of Physiology, Endocrinology and Metabolism, 285*, E363-E371.

McPherron, A. C., Lawler, A. M., & Lee, S. J. (1997). Regulation of skeletal muscle mass in mice by a new TGF-ß superfamily member. *Nature, 387*, 83-90.

McPherron, A. C., & Lee, S. J. (1997). Double muscling in Cattle due to mutations in the myostatin gene. *Proceedings of the National Academy of Sciences USA, 94*(23), 12457-12461.

Ménissier, F. (1982). Muscle hypertrophy of genetic origin and its use to improve beef production. In J. W. B. King & F. Ménissier (Eds.), *The Hague*. Nijhoff: The Netherlands.

Phillips, S., Tipton, K., Aarsland, A., Wolf, S., & Wolfe, R. (1997). Mixed muscle protein synthesis and breakdown after resistance exercise in humans. *American Journal of Physiology, Endocrinology and Metabolism, 273*, E99-E107.

Rasmussen, B. B., & Phillips, S. M. (2003). Contractile and nutritional regulation of human muscle growth. *Exercise and Sport Sciences Reviews, 31*(3), 127-131.

Reis, E., Frick, U., & Schmidtbleicher, D. (1995). Frequency variations of strength training sessions triggered by the phases of the menstrual cycle. *International Journal of Sports Medicine, 16*(8), 545-550.

Roth, S. M., Martel, G. F., Ferell, R. E., Metter, E. J., Hurley, B. F., & Rogers, M. A. (2003). Myostatin gene expression is reduced in humans with heavy-resistance strength training: A brief communication. *Experimental Biology and Medicine, 228*, 706-709.

Sallinen, J., Pakarinen, A., Ahtiainen, J., Kraemer, W. J., Volek, J. S., & Hakkinen, K. (2004). Relationship between diet and serum anabolic hormone responses to heavy-resistance exercise in men. *International Journal of Sports Medicine, 25*(8), 627-633.

Sharma, M., Langley, B., Bass, J., & Kambadur, R. (2001). Myostatin in muscle growth and repair. *Exercise and Sport Sciences Reviews, 29*(4), 155-158.

Sorichter, S., Puschendorf, B., & Mair, J. (1999). Skeletal muscle injury induced by eccentric muscle action: Muscle proteins as markers of muscle fibre injury. *Exercise Immunology Review, 5*, 5-21.

Viru, A., Smirnova, T., Karelson, K., Snegovskaya, V., & Viru, M. (1996). Determinants and modulators of hormonal responses to exercise. *Biology of Sport, 13*(3), 169-181.

Viru, M., Litvinova, L., Smirnova, T., & Viru, A. (1994). Glucocorticoids in metabolic control during exer-cise: Glycogen metabolism. *The Journal of Sports Medicine and Physical Fitness, 34*(4), 377-382.

Volek, J. S., Kraemer, W. J., Bush, J. A., Incledon, T., & Boetes, M. (1997). Testosterone and cortisol in relationship to dietary nutrients and resistance exercise. *Journal of Applied Physiology, 82*(1), 49-54.

Walker, K. S., Kambadur, R., Sharma, M., & Smith, H. K. (2004). Resistance training alters plasma myostatin but not IGF-1 in healthy men. *Medicine & Science in Sports & Exercise, 36*(5), 787-793.

Wehling, M., Cai, B., & Tidball, G. (2000). Modulation of myostatin expression during modified muscle use. *Federation of the American Societies of Experimental Biology Journal, 14*, 103-110.

Willoughby, D. S., Sultemeire, S., & Brown, M. (2003). Human disuse atrophy after 28 days in a lower-limb walking boot: A case study. *Journal of Exercise Physiology online, 6*(2), 88-96.

Willoughby, D. S., & Taylor, L. (2004a). Effects of concentric and eccentric muscle actions on serum myostatin and follistatin-like related gene levels. *Journal of Sports Science and Medicine, 39,*(3), 226-233.

Willoughby, D. S., & Taylor, L. (2004b). Effects of sequential bouts of resistance exercise on androgen receptor expression. *Medicine & Science in Sports & Exercise, 36*(9), 1499-1506.

DWAYNE MASSEY

An analysis of full range of motion vs. partial range of motion training in the development of strength

Keywords: range of motion, partial range of motion, strength training, intensity, repetition

Introduction and literature review

Those involved in the pursuit of weight training to develop strength and lean muscle mass have long utilized partial range of motion training to meet these objectives. A partial range of motion repetition is defined as one that is completed in a restricted portion of the total lift. The area that will be the focus of our interest and the one that has suggested the most potential in the aforementioned areas is the completion of a repetition in the top or upper portion of a respective lift. For the bench press this would be considered the final 2 - 5 inches of the lift prior to full extension of the elbows (Graves, Pollock, Jones, Colvin, & Leggett, 1989; Lander, Bates, Sawhill, & Hamill, 1985; Mookerjee & Ratamess, 1999; Sisco & Little, 1997; Wilson, Elliott, & Kerr, 1989). In the squat, a partial repetition could be described as a half or quarter squat well above the parallel depth angle traditional advocated by most weight training experts. When applied to the standing barbell curl this technique would be performed in the final 3 - 4 inches of the curl movement or the upper portion of the lift. Due to the fact that heavier weights can be utilized through the restricted range of motion, training loads exceeding 100 % of a person's one repetition have been demonstrated (Mookerjee & Ratamess, 1999).

This training technique has ample antidotal and theoretical support in the strength and conditioning literature. Strength and conditioning experts in the former Soviet Union and eastern bloc countries have long purported this method of training as being vastly superior to full range of motion movements in many training and sporting contexts. However, it has only been relatively recently that scientific interest in this mode of training has been demonstrated by western scholars (Graves et al., 1989; Mookerjee & Ratamess, 1999; Sullivan, Knowlton, Devita, & Brown, 1996). A limited but growing portion of this research appears to support the premise that, at least as far as muscular strength is concerned, their maybe some practical benefits derived from partial range of motion training (cf. Graves et al., 1992; Graves et al., 1989; Jones, Hunter, Fleisig, Escamilla, & Lemak, 1999; Massey, Vincent, Maneval, Moore, & Johnson, 2004; Mookerjee & Ratamess, 1999; Sullivan et al., 1996).

Sisco and Little (1997) make numerous assertions related to this area of inquiry. These authors support the premise that utilizing heavy weights through an individual's strongest range of motion is vastly superior to full range of motion movements in the development of muscular strength and size. The authors cite several reasons for their beliefs. These include:

- Training with weights in the person's strongest range of motion significantly increases the overload experienced by the body.
- Overload is the single most important variable to be manipulated in determining the overall progress obtained from a resistance training program.
- Partial repetitions provide superior overload as compared to full range of motion movement due to the mechanical advantage provided and the consequentially greater weight that can be lifted through the person's strongest range of motion.
- The ability over time to handle greater weight causes an adaptation response by the body which ultimately produces larger and stronger muscles.
- A precursor to being able to lift heavy weights is the development of strong ligaments and tendons. Partial repetitions are portrayed as the supreme method of training for achieving this result.
- Partial repetitions are characterized as being more specific to everyday activities and sport applications. The point is made that when we push a car that has run out of gas we do so with our arms outstretched and our legs assisting in the movement. When an offensive lineman makes a block in American football this is also performed in a limited range of motion fashion. Because partial range of motion movements are more specific to these real world activities there is considered to be some carryover effect that enhance the performance of these activities.

Sisco and Little (1997) make an interesting argument in support of their position. They back up their assertions with convincing anecdotal information and the testimonials of famous strong men. However, the research data that present to substantiate their claims is limited.

Wilson (1994) agreed with many of the assertions made by Sisco and Little (1997). He similarly maintains that the nature of the overload imposed on the muscles is the most important factor determining gains obtained from a resistance training program. He agrees that partial range of motion training provides a greater overload than full range of motion exercise, thereby causing a superior adaptation effect, which over time causes the musculature of the body to grow and get stronger. Wilson (1994), as were Sisco and Little (1997), is convinced that the more the training protocol and the athletic activity resemble each other the higher the probability that a positive transference in performance will occurs. He argues emphatically that partial range of motion exercise is more likely to produce this transference. Wilson (1994) utilizes the comparison of the full and half squat to illustrate his point. He states that with the full squat the amount of weight that can be lifted is limited by the force that can be generated to overcome the "sticking point". In the squat this has been found between the joint angles of 95 and 115 degrees. Once through this region the lift becomes comparatively easier to complete. In fact, between the joint angles 140 - 180 degrees a weight needed to get through the sticking point is not sufficient to provide to an overload stimulus at this upper portion of the range of motion. However, at the same time the stimulus at these joint angles is insufficient, the actually ability of the body to create force is one and a half times greater than at the region of the sticking point (95 - 115 degrees). The consequence of this, according to Wilson (1994), is that in the area of greatest force production and in which most athletic skills are demonstrated, the musculature of the body is nowhere near loaded to its full potential.

On the other hand, a half squat movement is represented as meeting this criterion. By lifting super maximal weights the high levels of force necessary to maximize training gains within this important range of motion can be realized (McLaughlin, Gillman, & Lardner, 1977).

Another important consequence cited by Wilson (1994) related to the use of the partial movement is that of disinhibition. The human body has built in safeguards that operate to prevent the production of excessive force. When the central nervous system perceives the tension within the body is too high it sends an inhibitory signal to the individual motor units causing the muscles to shut down preventing further force production. This mechanism serves a protective function which operates to keep the body from injuring itself. By utilizing a heavier weight then could normal be lifted, the over sensitivity of this protective mechanism is over time reduced, allowing the individual to get nearer to their absolute maximum force producing capabilities.

As mentioned earlier the former Soviet Union and Eastern Bloc countries were convinced of the value of partial range of motion training. In fact, Zatsiorsky (1995), an architect of the Soviet's success in Olympic and international competition identifies this method of training as being the most popular exercise strategy among superior athletes within these former regimes. Referred to as the accentuation principle, Zatsiorsky (1995) features this concept prominently in his popular book published in the west entitled the Science and Practice of Strength Training. He insists that strength training should be performed in the range of the main sport movement where the demand for high force production is maximal. Also using the squat to make clear his position, Zatsiorsky (1995) compares elite volleyball players and ski jumpers. He states that the majority of squat training for a volleyball player should consist of a semi-squat movement due to the volleyball player performing their leaps in the air from a crouched position. The ski jumper on the other hand who travels down and takes off from a ramp in a squat position should perform the majority of their training with a deeper squatting motion.

Limited range of motion exercise has long been utilized in rehabilitation programs to overcome injuries and increase overall range of motion strength. To investigate the utility of this training technique, Graves et al. (1989) conducted training on a Nautilus knee extension machine. The researchers divided subjects into three training groups. One group trained with a full range of motion, and two additional groups trained at different restricted ranges of motion within that full range of motion. A separate group served as a control. Isometric measurements were utilized at eight sites along the full range of motion to determine strength gains during the investigation. Subjects were both pre and post tested. The findings indicated while strength gains were greatest in the areas in which training took place all of the training groups improved in isometric strength at each of the sites measured when compared with a control group.

Graves et al. (1992) followed up this first study with a second one focusing on the use of limited range of motion resistance exercise to improve lumbar extension strength. Training was conducted on a lumbar extension machine using a similar protocol. The findings of this study were even more dramatic than the previous investigation. As before, strength gains for the limited range of motion groups were greatest in the range of motion trained. However, no statistical differences in strength were noted at the conclusion of the study between any of the training groups at any of the sites measured ($p > 0.05$).

Sullivan et al. (1996) investigated whether restricted range of motion weight training exercise would accentuate the cardiovascular response compared to full range of motion movements. Training was conducted using the barbell curl exercise. The researchers found that the restricted range of motion exercise produced significantly increased heart rate, blood PH and lactate levels, and rate of perceived exertion as compared to the full range of motion movements. A biomechanical analysis conducted in conjunction with this study indicated that greater torque was produced by the restricted range of motion exercise as opposed to the full range of motion movement. The researchers theorized that the restricted range of motion increased the rate of movement, thereby increasing the work performed for a given period of time, resulting in a greater training effect.

Mookerjee and Ratamess (1999) investigated strength differences following an acute exposure to full and partial range of motion bench press exercise. Subjects were tested on the 1-RM and the 5-RM, for both the partial and full range of motion movements, separated by a period of four days. The results of the study indicated that the partial range of motion performance increased significantly for both the 1-RM and the 5-RM while no such improvement was observed for the full range of motion movement. The researchers contended that this improvement might have occurred due to a motor learning response and improved coordination of both primary and stabilizing muscles involved in the activity.

The researchers hypothesized that those individuals who trained exclusively with a full range of motion might fail to optimally train in the area where maximal force development occurs. They speculated that partial range of motion exercise allows optimal force production to occur due to elimination of the sticking point, thus giving the lifter a biomechanical advantage. The researchers based this conclusion on the fact that subjects were able to use greater loads in the partial movements than in the full range of motion movements. These findings seem to support Sullivan et al. (1996) who reported greater torque production during performance of partial range of motion barbell curls.

Partial range of motion training was incorporated into Jones et al. (1999) investigation utilizing the bench press to determine the effects of maximum concentric acceleration of the barbell as compared to traditional bench press technique on the development of strength and power. The subjects participating in this study were NCAA Division IAA football players. One partial range of motion set was incorporated into the program for both groups. The partial set was performed in the same fashion as the full range of motion sets for each of these individual groups. Findings related to this study indicated that the maximum concentric acceleration group demonstrated significantly greater increases in strength and power than did the training movements performed at the slower training speed. Since the partial movements were included in both training protocols it could not be determined if the partial repetitions played a role in the improvements found for the acceleration group. However, the researchers recommended since evidence suggested a possible link future investigation were needed focusing more specifically on this method of training.

Methods

Upon scrutiny it becomes clear that the research done involving partial range of motion exercise, while provocative, has several limitations. Most of our orientation related to this technique is heavily influenced by hear say, testimonials by those who purported having success utilizing the technique, and those proponents of this form of training who back up their claims with limited empirical data. Other limitations related to these previous investigations include limited training protocols, research involving only a small number of subjects, the partial technique being only a minor aspect of the research and not the primary focus of the study, and the length of training time involved being of extremely short duration. Due to the limited scope of the research previously conducted in this area, Massey et al. (2004) decided to conduct a study to better elucidate the partial technique's place in an overall training regimen.

This investigation covered a 10-week period using the bench press as the criterion measurement. Subjects in this study consisted of male college students participating in university weight lifting classes. Subjects were classified as recreational weightlifters having some experience in the activity of weight training. These individuals ranged from those who worked out frequently at moderately high levels of intensity to those who worked out occasionally or infrequently. Those involved in intercollegiate athletics or bodybuilding, or who reported use of performance enhancing drugs were excluded.

These subjects were divided into three groups. Group 1 (N = 11) trained with 3 full range of motion sets on the bench press. Group 2 (N = 15) trained with 3 partial range of motion sets. As delineated earlier for our purposes a partial range of motion repetition was defined as one that is beyond the sticking point 2 - 5 inches from full extension of the elbows. Group 3 (N = 30) trained with a

combination of partial and full range of motion sets. To equalize these two combinations Group 3 performed 2 partial range of motion sets and 1 full range of motion set for the first 5 weeks. For the next 5 weeks this regimen was reversed and the subjects performed 1 partial range of motion set and 2 full range of motion sets. Supervisory personnel who conducted the training were all instructed in the training protocol prior to the investigation.
Training sessions were conducted two days per week. All bench press protocols incorporated three sets of fifteen repetitions. When subjects completed the prescribed number of sets and repetitions on any of the exercises performed in the study, they were allowed to increase the weight by five pounds in the next training session. Beginning weight for the bench press was determined by a 1-RM as prescribed by Baechle, Earle and Wathen (2000). The full range of motion group initially trained with sets of 65 % of their 1-RM. The partial range of motion group began the study training with sets at 100 % of their 1-RM. In addition to being tested at the beginning of the study, subjects were also post-tested on the 1-RM at the end of the tenth week. This test has been found to have a reliability of 0.93 (Johnson & Nelson, 1974). Except for the bench press, all subjects engaged in the same training routine during the duration of the investigation (cf. table 1).

Table 1: Training routine

exercise	set	repetitions
squat	3	10
upright row	3	15
standing curl	3	10
lat pulldown	3	10
crunches	3	15
leg curls	3	12
calf raises	3	12

Subjects were not allowed to do any other weight training activities outside of the perimeters of the study. A 2/4 format was used to perform the full range of motion repetitions. The weight was lowered in four seconds and raised in two seconds (Brzycki, 1995). Due to the restricted nature of the partial range of motion repetitions the individual's natural lifting speed was utilized. A rest period of 2 minutes was permitted between sets (Brzycki, 1995).

Statistical data

Statistical analysis of data obtain consisted of two methods. A t-test was utilized to determine differences within each of the groups' post treatment. Due to pre-test variations between groups on the 1-RM, a univariate analysis of covariance (ANCOVA) was utilized to assess differences between the three groups' post treatment. Statistical significance on both analyses was identified as being at a Bonferroni corrected $p \leq 0.0125$ level.

Results

The results of these analysis indicated that the 1-RM for each of the three groups increased from pre to post test. The t-test indicated that the increase for each of the groups was statistically significant (cf. table 2), with the full and partial range of motion experiencing almost identical mean increases of 25 and 24.33 pounds respectively, and the combination group experiencing an increase of 16.50 pounds. The ANCOVA found no differences between the groups post treatment (cf. table 3).

Table 2: Paired sample correlations for 1-RM on the bench press

				group = full				
		mean	N	std.	std. error	t	df	sig.
pair 1	pre	166.36	11	44.16	13.31	-5.52	10	< .001
	post	191.36	11	47.12	14.20			
				group = partial				
		mean	N	std.	std. error	t	df	sig.
pair 1	pre	176.00	15	44.36	11.45	-7.13	14	< .001
	post	200.33	15	47.52	12.27			
				group = mixed				
		mean	N	std.	std. error	t	df	sig.
pair 1	pre	205.50	30	59.02	10.77	-6.98	29	< .001
	post	222.00	30	57.18	10.44			

Table 3: Tests of between-subject effects (ANCOVA)

source	type III sum of squares	df	mean squares	F	sig.
corrected model	148783.37		49594.45	273.92	< 0.001
intercept	3064.07	1	3064.07	16.92	< .0001
pre	139243.03	1	139243.03	769.06	< 0.001
group	634.64	2	317.32	1.75	0.183
error	9414.84	52	181.05		
total	2632000.00	56			
corrected total	158198.21	55			

Discussion

The findings of this investigation are interesting. If the hypothesis that overload is the single most important determinant involved in strength development is correct, then one would anticipate that those who engage in partial repetition training should experience the greatest levels of strength development. This was not a finding of this investigation. In fact, no discernable strength differences were found between any of the three groups at the conclusion of the study. Most traditional experts in the field have long held that partial repetitions provide no benefit to the serious weight lifter. Again, this was not the finding of this investigation, at least as far as the development of maximal strength was concerned. Partial and mixed repetitions were found to be equally as effective as full repetitions within the perimeters of this study.

At least two rival hypotheses can be drawn from these findings. First, if partial range of motion training cannot be demonstrated to be superior to full range of motion training why not advocate full repetitions? The argument has always been that the benefits of increased flexibility and decreased susceptibility to injury provided by full range of motion repetitions preclude the use of partial range of motion repetitions as a practical training option. The second possible hypothesis is if partial range of motion training is just as effective as full range of motion training; why not advocate the partial technique as a supplement or aid in overcoming training plateaus or as an adjunct to full range of motion training. This research appears to give some support to the adherents who support the viability of this training option.

The role that heavier weights associated with the partial range of motion technique play in strength increases through a full range of motion was not completely discerned from this investigation. However, due to the length of the study, gains in muscle mass from the training protocol could be expected to contribute only minimally to the strength increases observed (Brandenburg & Docherty, 2002; Brzycki, 1995; Komi, 1986). This supports Wilson (1994) contention that a strong neuromuscular adaptation is associated with the partial technique, and that it can positively influence strength over the full range of motion. It does appear beyond question that, at the very least, training at the top end of the training movement does increase strength within that specific range of motion (Graves et al., 1992; Graves et al., 1989; Lander et al., 1985; Wilson, 1994). Such an effect would appear to be of benefit to a power lifter as they attempt to lock a weight out at the top of the lift. Similarly, other athletes who must demonstrate strength in the upper portion of their range of motion would also seem to benefit from the partial range of motion technique. This reasoning suggests support for those researchers that assert utilizing partial range of motion exercise in addition to more traditional weight training practices assists the individual to reach their maximum strength potential (Mookerjee & Ratamess, 1999; Wilson, 1994; Zatsiorsky, 1995).

After analysis the Massey et al. (2004) study provides additional evidence in support of partial range of motion training as a viable training option. Multiple research studies now indicate that the partial range of motion technique can have a positive influence on overall range of motion strength (Graves et al., 1992; Graves et al., 1989; Lander et al., 1985; Massey et al., 2004). While there remains some question of its proper place in an overall training regimen, it does appear that strength and conditioning professions can, with some measure of confidence, incorporate the partial technique into their overall training program as an adjunct or change up to their regular training prescriptions. However, further research is needed to elucidate the place of partial range of motion exercise in an overall training regimen. Further investigations should be conducted with different populations, different training exercises, larger N sizes, and longer training periods.

While it may ultimately be demonstrated that this technique has only limited applications, further scrutiny may continue to yield surprising findings. The body of literature amassed to date on this subject leads to speculation that advanced weight lifters, being accustomed to pushing themselves closer to their physiological limits, may be in an even more advantageous position to benefit from the partial technique. Also, a person who has been training with weights for a longer period of time and has reached a plateau where little or no increases in strength are occurring may also be in a better position to benefit from partial range of motion training. Not until additional comprehensive investigations are conducted will we be able to answer these questions with any degree of appropriate justification.

References

Baechle, T. R., Earle, R., & Wathen, D. (2000). Resistance training. In T. R. Baechle & R. Earle (Eds.), *Essentials of strength training and conditioning* (pp. 395-425). Champaign, IL: Human Kinetics.

Brandenburg, J. P., & Docherty, D. (2002). The effects of accentuated eccentric loading on strength, muscle hypertrophy, and neural adaptations in trained individuals. *Journal of Strength and Conditioning Research, 16*(1), 25-32.

Brzycki, M. (1995). *A practical approach to strength training* (3rd ed.). Lincolnwood, IL: Masters Press.

Graves, J., Pollock, M., Leggett, S., Carpenter, D., Fix, C., & Fulton, M. (1992). Limited range-of-motion lumbar extension strength training. *Medicine & Science in Sports & Exercise, 24*(1), 128-133.

Graves, J., Pollock, M. L., Jones, A. E., Colvin, A. B., & Leggett, S. H. (1989). Specificity of limited range of motion variable resistance training. *Medicine & Science in Sports & Exercise, 21*(1), 84-89.

Johnson, B., & Nelson, J. (1974). *Practical measurements for evaluation in physical education*. Minneapolis, MN: Burgess Publishing Company.

Jones, K., Hunter, G., Fleisig, G., Escamilla, R., & Lemak, L. (1999). The effects of compensatory acceleration on upper-body strenght and power in collegiate football players. *Journal of Strength and Conditioning Research, 13*(2), 99-105.

Komi, P. V. (1986). Training of muscle strength and power: Interaction of neuromotoric, hypertropic, and mechanical factors. *International Journal of Sports Medicine, 7*(1), S10-15.

Lander, J. E., Bates, B. T., Sawhill, J. A., & Hamill, J. (1985). A comparison between freeweigth and isokinetic bench pressing. *Medicine & Science in Sports & Exercise, 17*(3), 344-353.

Massey, C. D., Vincent, J., Maneval, M., Moore, M., & Johnson, J. T. (2004). An analysis of full range of motion vs. partial range of motion training in the development of strength in untrained men. *Journal of Strength and Conditioning Research, 18*(3), 518-521.

McLaughlin, T., Gillman, C., & Lardner, T. (1977). A kinetic model of performance in the parallel squat by champion powerlifters. *Medicine and Science in Sports, 9*(2), 128-133.

Mookerjee, S., & Ratamess, N. (1999). Comparison of strenght differences and joint action durations between full and partial range-of-motion bench press exercise. *Journal of Strength and Conditioning Research, 13*(1), 76-81.

Sisco, P., & Little, J. (1997). *Power factor training: A scientific approach to building lean muscle mass*. Chicago, IL: Contemporary Books.

Sullivan, J., Knowlton, R., Devita, P., & Brown, D. (1996). Cardiovascular response to restricted range of motion resistance exercise. *Journal of Strength and Conditioning Research, 10*(1), 3-7.

Wilson, G. (1994). Strength and power in sports. In J. Bloomfield, T. Ackland & B. Elliott (Eds.), *Applied anatomy and biomechanics in sports* (pp. 110-208). Boston: Blackwell Scientific Publications.

Wilson, G., Elliott, B., & Kerr, G. (1989). Bar path and force profile characteristics for maximal and sub-maximal loads in the bench press. *International Journal of Sport Biomechanics, 5*,(4), 390-402.

Zatsiorsky, V. M. (1995). *Science and practice of strength training*. Champaign, IL: Human Kinetics.

Index

R

S

T

W

Directory of the authors

Bishop, Mark D., Dr., Department of Physical Therapy, University of Florida, Gainesville, Florida 32610-0154, USA
email: mbishop@phhp.ufl.edu

Emrich, Eike, Prof. Dr., Johann Wolfgang Goethe-Universität Frankfurt/Main, Ginnheimer Landstraße 39, 60487 Frankfurt am Main, Germany
email: e.emrich@sport.uni-frankfurt.de

Engelke, Klaus, PD Dr., Institut für Medizinische Physik, Friedrich Alexander Universität Erlangen-Nürnberg, Henkestraße 91, 91052 Erlangen, Germany
email: klaus@imp.uni-erlangen.de

Eifler, Christoph, Dipl. Sportlehrer, BSA-Akademie u. Private Berufsakademie, Hermann Neuberger Sportschule, 66123 Saarbrücken, Germany
email: c-eifler@bsa-akademie.de

Ferrauti, Alexander, Prof. Dr., Ruhr-Universität Bochum, Fakultät für Sportwissenschaft, Stiepeler Straße 129, 44801 Bochum, Germany
email: alexander.ferrauti@rub.de

Freiwald, Jürgen, Prof. Dr., Bergische Universität Wuppertal, Gaußstraße 20, 42119 Wuppertal, Germany
email: freiwald@uni-wuppertal.de

Fröhlich, Michael, Dr., Olympiastützpunkt Rheinland-Pfalz/Saarland, c/o Hermann Neuberger Sportschule, Geb. 56, 66123 Saarbrücken, Germany
email: m.froehlich@olympiastuetzpunkt.org

Gießing, Jürgen, Dr. Dr., Philipps-Universität Marburg, Wilhelm-Röpke-Straße 6 B, 35032 Marburg, Germany
email: giessing@staff.uni-marburg.de

Glass, Stephen C., Prof. Dr., Department of Movement Science, Grand Valley State University, 1 Campus Drive, Allendale, MI 49401, USA
email: glassst@gvsu.edu

Greiwing, Andreas, Bergische Universität Wuppertal, Gaußstraße 20, 42119 Wuppertal, Germany
email: greiwing@uni-wuppertal.de

Goebel, Sven, Dr., Forschungsabteilung Kieser Training (FAKT), Neusser Straße 27-29, 50670 Köln, Germany
email: sven.goebel@kieser-training.com

Kaminski, Thomas W., Prof. Dr., Department of Health, Nutrition & Exercise Sciences, University of Delaware, Newark, DE 19716, USA
email: kaminski@udel.edu

Kemmler, Wolfgang, PD Dr., Osteoporose-Forschungszentrum, Institut für Medizinische Physik, Friedrich Alexander Universität Erlangen-Nürnberg, Henkestraße 91, 91052 Erlangen, Germany
email: wolfgang@imp.uni-erlangen.de

Klein, Markus, Dipl. Sportlehrer, Johann Wolfgang Goethe-Universität Frankfurt/Main, Ginnheimer Landstraße 39, 60487 Frankfurt, Germany
email: M.Klein@em.uni-frankfurt.de

Lauber, Dirk, Diplomsport-Ökonom, Institut für Sportwissenschaften und Sport, Friedrich Alexander Universität Erlangen-Nürnberg, Gebberstraße 123, 91054 Erlangen, Germany
email: DirkLauber@t-online.de

Lichtenegger, Niklas, Mag., University of sports sciences Graz, Mozartgasse 14, A-8010 Graz, Österreich,
email: n.l@nik-training.com

Massey, Dwayne, Dr., University of Southern Mississippi, School of Human Performance and Recreation, 118 College Drive 5142, Hattiesburg, MS, USA
email: DMassey@usm.edu

Müller, Andreas, Dr., Heinrich-Heine-Straße 70, 08412 Werdau, Germany
email: Andreas.Mller2@gmx.net

Preuss, Peter, Dipl. Sportlehrer, Rheinische Friedrich-Wilhelms-Universität Bonn, Nachtigallenweg 86, 53127 Bonn, Germany
email: peter.preuss@uni-bonn.de

Schmidtbleicher, Dietmar, Prof. Dr., Johann Wolfgang Goethe-Universität Frankfurt/Main, Ginnheimer Landstraße 39, 60487 Frankfurt/Main, Germany
email: schmidtbleicher@sport.uni-frankfurt.de

Stephan, Anika, Assistentin Leiter Forschungsabteilung Kieser Training (FAKT), Neusser Straße 27-29, 50670 Köln, Germany
email: anika.stephan@kieser-training.de

Remmert, Hubert, Dr., Ruhr-Universität Bochum, Fakultät für Sportwissenschaft, Stiepeler Straße 129, 44801 Bochum, Germany
email: hubert.remmert@rub.de

Schischek, Alexander, Dipl. Sportwissenschaftler, Ruhr-Universität Bochum, Fakultät für Sportwissenschaft, Stiepeler Straße 129, 44801 Bochum, Germany
email: schischek77@aol.com

Stanton, Douglas R., Dr., Human Performance Lab, Wayne State College, Wayne, NE., USA

Strack, Andreas, Dipl. Sportlehrer, BSA-Akademie u. Private Berufsakademie, Hermann Neuberger Sportschule, 66123 Saarbrücken, Germany
email: a-Strack@bsa-akademie.de

Von Stengel, Simon, Dr., Osteoporose-Forschungszentrum, Institut für Medizinische Physik, Friedrich Alexander Universität Erlangen-Nürnberg, Henkestraße 91, 91052 Erlangen, Germany
email: simon@imp.uni-erlangen.de

Zamhöfer, Tobias, Dipl. Sportwissenschaftler, Ruhr-Universität Bochum, Fakultät für Sportwissenschaft, Stiepeler Straße 129, 44801 Bochum, Germany
email: zami@surfeu.de